The CHAPTER <797> ANSWER BOOK

PATRICIA C. KIENLE

Director, Accreditation and Medication Safety

Cardinal Health
Innovative Delivery Solutions

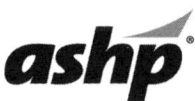

Any correspondence regarding this publication should be sent to the publisher, ASHP, 4500 East-West Highway, Suite 900, Bethesda, MD 20814, attention: Special Publishing.

The information presented herein reflects the opinions of the contributors and advisors. It should not be interpreted as an official policy of ASHP or as an endorsement of any product.

Because of ongoing research and improvements in technology, the information and its applications contained in this text are constantly evolving and are subject to the professional judgment and interpretation of the practitioner due to the uniqueness of a clinical situation. The editors and ASHP have made reasonable efforts to ensure the accuracy and appropriateness of the information presented in this document. However, any user of this information is advised that the editors and ASHP are not responsible for the continued currency of the information, for any errors or omissions, and/or for any consequences arising from the use of the information in the document in any and all practice settings. Any reader of this document is cautioned that ASHP makes no representation, guarantee, or warranty, express or implied, as to the accuracy and appropriateness of the information contained in this document and specifically disclaims any liability to any party for the accuracy and/or completeness of the material or for any damages arising out of the use or non-use of any of the information contained in this document.

Vice President, Publishing: Daniel Cobaugh

Editorial Project Manager, books and elearning Course: Ruth Bloom

Editorial Project Manager, Publications Production Center: Kristin Eckles

Cover & Page Design: David Wade

Editorial Consultant: Toni Fera, BS Pharm, PharmD

Library of Congress Cataloging-in-Publication Data

Names: Kienle, Patricia C., author. | American Society of Health-System Pharmacists, issuing body.
Title: The chapter <797> answer book / Patricia C. Kienle.
Other titles: United States pharmacopeia.
Description: Bethesda : ASHP, [2020] | Includes bibliographical references and index. | Summary: "The Chapter <797> Answer Book will provide a balance of both formal requirements of the USP chapter as well as practical advice and consideration in complying with the chapter. The Chapter <797> Answer Book will follow a sterile product from receipt to preparation in a healthcare facility, addressing core elements of the USP chapter. Each section will begin with a brief introduction, providing an overview of the key issues and requirements of the section. The overview will be followed by questions and answers, many from live overview sessions on <797>, covering the specifics of compliance"-- Provided by publisher.
Identifiers: LCCN 2019031909 (print) | ISBN 9781585286355 (paperback) | ISBN 9781585286362 (adobe pdf)
Subjects: MESH: Technology, Pharmaceutical--standards | Sterilization--standards | Drug Contamination--prevention & control | Pharmacopoeias as Topic | United States
Classification: LCC RS139 (print) | LCC RS139 (ebook) | NLM QV 778 | DDC --1/615.1dc23
LC record available at https://lccn.loc.gov/2019031909
LC ebook record available at https://lccn.loc.gov/2019031910

© 2020, American Society of Health-System Pharmacists, Inc. All rights reserved.

No part of this publication may be reproduced or transmitted in any form or by any means, electronic or mechanical, including photocopying, microfilming, and recording, or by any information storage and retrieval system, without written permission from the American Society of Health-System Pharmacists.

ASHP is a service mark of the American Society of Health-System Pharmacists, Inc.; registered in the U.S. Patent and Trademark Office.

ISBN: 978-1-58528-635-5

10 9 8 7 6 5 4 3 2 1

TABLE OF CONTENTS

Preface vii
Introduction ix
Acknowledgments/Reviewers xi
Acronyms xii
Disclaimer xiii
List of Questions xv
List of Exhibits xxxv
List of Tables xxxv
List of Boxes xxxvi

1. USP <797> Availability 1
2. General Principles of USP <797> 3
3. Contents of Sections of USP <797> 5
4. Scope of USP <797> 9
5. Human Resources 13
   5.1 *Designated Person* 13
   5.2 *Responsibilities of Compounding Personnel* 15
   5.3 *Documenting Competence* 15
   5.4 *Hazard Communication Plan* 16
6. Policies and Procedures 19
7. Garb and Hand Hygiene 23
   7.1 *General Information* 23
   7.2 *Hand Hygiene* 24
   7.3 *Gloves* 25
   7.4 *Gowns* 26
   7.5 *Hair Covers* 27
   7.6 *Masks* 27
   7.7 *Sleeves* 28
   7.8 *Shoe Covers* 28
   7.9 *Eye Protection* 28
   7.10 *Respiratory Protection* 29
   7.11 *Garbing Procedures* 29
8. Immediate Use and Preparation for Administration 33
9. Personnel Training and Competence Documentation 37
   9.1 *Initial Training* 37
   9.2 *Hand Hygiene* 41
   9.3 *Garbing* 42

TABLE OF CONTENTS (continued)

  9.4 *Gloved Fingertip and Thumb Test* 42
  9.5 *Aseptic Technique* 45
  9.6 *Media Fill Test* 46
  9.7 *Requalification* 49
10. Sterile Products and Supplies 51
  10.1 *General Information* 51
  10.2 *Use of Nonsterile Starting Components* 51
11. Facility Design, Engineering Controls, and Equipment 55
  11.1 *General Facility Design Information* 55
  11.2 *Storage Areas* 59
  11.3 *Primary Engineering Controls* 60
  11.4 *Secondary Engineering Controls—General Information* 61
  11.5 *Anterooms* 64
  11.6 *Presterilization Area for Weighing Powders* 67
  11.7 *Cleanroom Suites* 67
  11.8 *Segregated Compounding Areas for Nonhazardous CSPs* 69
  11.9 *Containment Segregated Compounding Areas for Hazardous CSPs* 70
  11.10 *Pass-Through Chambers* 71
  11.11 *Refrigerator and Freezer Placement* 73
  11.12 *Other Compounding Area Equipment* 74
  11.13 *Compounding Immediate-Use CSPs in Ambient Air* 75
  11.14 *Allergenic Extracts Compounding Area* 76
  11.15 *Segregated Radiopharmaceutical Processing Area* 77
12. Daily Nonviable Monitoring 79
13. Certification of Engineering Controls 83
14. Compounding 87
  14.1 *General Information* 87
  14.2 *Nonsterile-to-Sterile Compounding* 90
  14.3 *Master Formulation Records* 92
  14.4 *Compounding Records* 93
  14.5 *Allergenic Extracts* 95
  14.6 *Radiopharmaceuticals* 95
15. Beyond-Use Dates 99
  15.1 *General Beyond-Use Date Information* 99
  15.2 *Active Pharmaceutical Ingredients and Other Components* 106
  15.3 *Vial/Bag Systems* 107
  15.4 *Vials and Other Dosage Forms* 107
  15.5 *Compounded Stock Bags* 109
16. Dispensing and Packaging 111

TABLE OF CONTENTS (continued)

17. Cleaning and Disinfecting 113
    17.1   General Information *113*
    17.2   Types of Cleaning Solutions *117*
    17.3   Cleaning PECs and Other Compounding Equipment *118*
    17.4   Cleaning Compounding Areas *120*
    17.5   Cleaning Supplies Needed for Compounding *121*
18. Environmental Monitoring 123
    18.1   General Information *123*
    18.2   Active Air Sampling *126*
    18.3   Surface Sampling *128*
    18.4   Reacting to Out-of-Specification Results *131*
19. Quality Assurance and Quality Control 133
20. What Do I Do Now? 135

Future Editions 137
References 138
Index 141

PREFACE

The Chapter <797> Answer Book provides an explanation of elements of *USP <797> Sterile Preparations* and best practices to comply with the requirements and recommendations of the USP General Chapter.

The author is a member of the USP Compounding Expert Committee, but this publication is not endorsed by or affiliated with USP.

Comments in this book are related to USP <797>, *USP 42–NF 37, Second Revision*, 2019. Updates to those documents must be considered when designing policies and practices.

Patricia C. Kienle

Compounding IV Solutions in the 1930s

At that time [ca. 1930], [Dr. Harvey] Cushing's solution was formulated at each nursing unit by adding the contents of a powder pack, compounded individually in the hospital pharmacy, to a liter of boiling distilled water. After it cooled, the solution was poured into a burette and administered intravenously through used rubber tubing and a glass adapter affixed to a needle. The burette and tubing were sterilized by boiling in an instrument sterilizer. On wards that had a bedpan sterilizer, that was used. The glass burettes were stained and often opaque and sticky. In the operating room and in a cleaner context, nurse-anesthetists prepared and administered 5% dextrose in Cushing's solution, but reactions were masked by anesthesia.

— Walter CW. Finding a better way. *JAMA*. 1990; 263:1675-8.

INTRODUCTION

Information concerning compounding has been incorporated in the *United States Pharmacopeia* since the first publication in 1820. Specific guidance for sterile compounding is provided in *USP General Chapter <797> Pharmaceutical Compounding—Sterile Preparations* and has evolved as contemporary practice requires the following:

- Originated as *USP General Chapter <1206> Sterile Drug Products for Home Use*
- First published as *USP General Chapter <797> Pharmaceutical Compounding—Sterile Preparations* in 2004
- Revised in 2008
- Published for public comment in 2015
- Public comments incorporated into second public comment version in 2018.
- Public comments incorporated and revised in 2019[1]

Pharmacies and other entities where sterile compounding occurs should obtain a copy of the full document. It is available from the United States Pharmacopeial Convention (USP), either as a part of the full *USP–NF* (National Formulary), or as part of the *USP Compounding Compendium*.

The USP is recognized in the Federal Food, Drug, and Cosmetic Act as an official compendium.[2] Numbering of the chapters is significant:

- USP chapters numbered below <1000> are considered applicable when they are referenced in a *General Notice*, a monograph, or in another general chapter numbered below <1000>.
- General Chapters numbered above <1000> are informational.
- Note that some regulatory agencies also consider those chapters above <1000> as requirements.

USP is a standard-setting organization, not a regulatory or enforcement agency. Regulatory bodies (such as the Centers for Medicare & Medicaid Services [CMS], state boards of pharmacy, state departments of health) and accreditation organizations enforce USP standards and/or include them in their standards.

In addition to USP <797>, other USP General Chapters also deal with compounding, including the following:

- *<795> Pharmaceutical Compounding—Nonsterile Preparations*
- *<800> Hazardous Drugs—Handling in Healthcare Settings*
- *<825> Radiopharmaceutical—Preparation, Compounding, Dispensing, and Repackaging*
- *<1066> Physical Environments That Promote Safe Medication Use*

INTRODUCTION (continued)

- *<1160> Pharmaceutical Calculations in Pharmacy Practice*
- *<1163> Quality Assurance in Pharmaceutical Compounding*
- *<1168> Compounding for Phase 1 Investigational Studies*
- *<1176> Prescription Balances and Volumetric Apparatus Used in Compounding*

Other USP General Chapters provide more specific information needed when certain types of compounded sterile preparations (CSPs) are mixed or to address compounding processes, including the following:

- *<7> Labeling*
- *<51> Antimicrobial Effectiveness Testing*
- *<71> Sterility Tests*
- *<85> Bacterial Endotoxins Test*
- *<659> Packaging and Storage Requirements*
- *<1085> Guidelines on Endotoxins Tests*
- *<1113> Microbial Characterization, Identification, and Strain Typing*
- *<1116> Microbial Control and Monitoring of Aseptic Processing Environments*
- *<1197> Good Distribution Practices for Bulk Pharmaceutical Excipients*
- *<1223> Validation of Alternative Microbial Methods*
- *<1228> Depyrogenation*
- *<1229> Sterilization of Compendial Articles*

References

1. United States Pharmacopeial Convention (USP). USP general chapter <797> hazardous drugs—handling in healthcare settings. In: *USP 42–NF 37*. Second Revision. Rockville, MD: USP; 2019.
2. United States Code, Title 21, §321, http://uscode.house.gov/view.xhtml?req=%28official+compendium%29+AND+%28%28title%3A%2821%29%29%29&f=treesort&fq=true&num=0&hl=true&edition=prelim&granuleId=USC-prelim-title21-section321 (accessed 2019 May 18).

ACKNOWLEDGMENTS

Current and past members of the USP Compounding Expert Committee devoted countless volunteer hours to discussion and development of practices that make patients and healthcare personnel safer. Many thanks to them, to Kate Douglass, and to USP staff Richard Schnatz, Jeanne Sun, Tiffany Chan, and Abbey Ammerman.

REVIEWERS

Kevin Hansen, PharmD, MS, BCPS

Assistant Director of Pharmacy
Moses H. Cone Memorial Hospital
Greensboro, North Carolina

Brenda Jensen, CPhT, CNMT, MBA

Pharmacy Technician
Compounding Consultants, LLC
Sioux Falls, South Dakota

Fred Massoomi, RPh, PharmD, FASHP

Senior Director
Hospital and Health-System Pharmacy Services
Visante
Omaha, Nebraska

ACRONYMS

ACD	automated compounding device
ACPH	air changes per hour
ACS	American Chemical Society
AECA	allergenic extracts compounding area
API	active pharmaceutical ingredient
APIC	Association for Professionals in Infection Control and Epidemiology
ASHP	American Society of Health-System Pharmacists
ASTM	American Society for Testing and Materials
BPS	Board of Pharmacy Specialties
BSC	biological safety cabinet
BUD	beyond-use date
C-SCA	containment segregated compounding area
CACI	compounding aseptic containment isolator
CAG	certification application guide
CAI	compounding aseptic isolator
CDC	Centers for Disease Control and Prevention
CETA	Controlled Environment Testing Association
CFU	colony-forming unit
CNBT	CETA National Board of Testing
CoA	certificate of analysis
CR	compounding record
CSP	compounded sterile preparation
CVE	containment ventilated enclosure
EM	environmental monitoring
FD&C Act	Food, Drug, & Cosmetic Act
FDA	U.S. Food and Drug Administration
HD	hazardous drug
HEPA	high-efficiency particulate air
ISO	International Standards Organization
LTC	long-term care
MEA	malt extract agar
MFR	master formulation record
NF	National Formulary
NIOSH	National Institute for Occupational Safety and Health
NRC	Nuclear Regulatory Commission
OSHA	Occupational Safety and Health Administration
PBP	pharmacy bulk package
PEC	primary engineering control
PNSU	probability of nonsterile unit
PPE	personal protective equipment
PTCB	Pharmacy Technician Accreditation Board
QA	quality assurance

ACRONYMS (continued)

QC	quality control
RABS	restricted-access barrier system
RAM License	radioactive materials license
SCA	segregated compounding area
SDA	Sabouraud dextrose agar
SDS	safety data sheet; formerly called material safety data sheet (MSDS)
SEC	secondary engineering control
sIPA	sterile 70% isopropyl alcohol
SOP	standard operating procedure
SRPA	segregated radiopharmaceutical processing area
TPN	total parenteral nutrition
TSA	trypticase soy agar
USP	United States Pharmacopeial Convention *United States Pharmacopeia*
wc	water column

Unless otherwise noted, compounding discussed in this text refers to nonhazardous sterile compounding.

DISCLAIMER

This book is based on the 2019 revision of USP <797>. In September 2019, USP announced that the 2019 revision had been appealed and that the 2008 version of USP <797> will remain in effect until the appeals process is resolved.

The 2019 revision of USP <797> expands explanatory information and updates many requirements. The following chart provides an overview of the major changes:

Topic	2008 Version	2019 Revision
Risk categories	Low, medium, and high	Elimination of this distinction
Categories of compounded sterile preparations (CSPs)		Category 1 and Category 2, based on the facility in which the CSP is mixed
Administration	Administration and preparation per manufacturer's labeling included in description of simple compounding	Administration and preparation per manufacturer's labeling is out of scope of <797> as long as it is intended for a single patient and will not be stored
Personnel		Requirement for designated person
Facility design	Allowance for placement of containment primary engineering controls (C-PECs) outside of negative pressure if only a low volume of hazardous drugs (HDs) compounded	Elimination of this exemption, because all HD compounding (unless exempted in the Assessment of Risk) must occur in negative pressure room
Placement of compounding aseptic isolator (CAI) outside of cleanroom suite	Allowance for full beyond-use dates (BUDs)	Full BUDs can only be assigned if the CAI is placed in a compliant compounding suite
BUDs in a segregated compounding area (SCA)	Maximum of 12 hours	Maximum of 12 hours room temperature or 24 hours refrigerated
BUDs	See details in chapter	See details in chapter, including limitations
Documentation		Master formulation records and compounding records required
Surface sampling	Required periodically	Required monthly

Because the 2019 revision includes contemporary best practices as well as current regulations, the reader is encouraged to comply with the 2019 revision, noting the regulatory differences that are presented.

LIST OF QUESTIONS

SECTION 1: USP <797> AVAILABILITY

1.1	Where can I find the full text of <797>?
1.2	When did <797> become official?
1.3	Why is there a need for a chapter on sterile compounding? Is this all about the meningitis scare from 2012?
1.4	Is <797> a guideline? A requirement?
1.5	How can <797> be a minimum standard if my state hasn't incorporated it into regulations?

SECTION 2: GENERAL PRINCIPLES OF USP <797>

2.1	Is this a new USP chapter?
2.2	What are the major differences between the version of <797> that has been official for a while and the 2019 version of <797>?
2.3	When must I comply with <797>?
2.4	What is the distinction between the terms *must* and *should* in the text of <797>?
2.5	If I'm just repackaging sterile products into unit doses, do I need to comply with <797>?
2.6	Are hazardous drugs addressed in <797>?
2.7	Are radiopharmaceuticals addressed in <797>?
2.8	Are allergens addressed in <797>?

SECTION 3: CONTENTS OF SECTIONS OF USP <797>

No questions

SECTION 4: SCOPE OF USP <797>

4.1	Who has to comply with <797>?
4.2	I've heard <797> referred to as a guideline and a standard. Which is correct? What's the difference?
4.3	Is <797> a regulation?
4.4	Does <797> apply to animals?
4.5	Can I select certain sections of <797> to be compliant with?
4.6	Is <797> in effect now?
4.7	What are examples of preparations that must comply—and those that do not comply—with <797>?
4.8	Does <797> apply to all compounds?
4.9	Does <797> apply to investigational agents?
4.10	I work in a hospital pharmacy. Do I need to comply with <795> or <797>?
4.11	Does <800> replace <797>?
4.12	Do community or mail-order pharmacies have to comply with <797>? How about a private physician's office?
4.13	Do pharmaceutical manufacturers have to comply with <797>?
4.14	Does a nursing home have to comply with <797>?
4.15	What types of activities aren't considered compounding?
4.16	How is administering medications distinguished from compounding?
4.17	I thought medications had to be administered within 1 hour of compounding. Which is correct: within 1 hour or within 4 hours?

LIST OF QUESTIONS (continued)

4.18	Does <797> include prepackaging from a vial to a unit-dose syringe?
4.19	<795> says repackaging is out of scope. Why is it included in <797>?
4.20	Is it OK to compound a preparation that can be mixed cheaper than the commercial product?
4.21	Who will enforce <797> for compliance outside of pharmacy settings?

SECTION 5: HUMAN RESOURCES

5.1	**Designated Person**
5.1-1	Who is the designated person mentioned in <797>?
5.1-2	Can the designated person be a committee instead of an individual?
5.1-3	Does the designated person need to be a pharmacist?
5.1-4	Does the designated person need to be a manager?
5.1-5	Is the designated person responsible for compliance with <797>?
5.1-6	Does oversight of sterile compounding have to be the designated person's sole job responsibility?
5.1-7	Can the designated person be responsible for more than one site?
5.1-8	Where can the designated person obtain the necessary training for this job?
5.1-9	How much training does the designated person need to have?
5.1-10	What types of activities is the designated person typically responsible for?
5.1-11	Does the designated person need to be board-certified?
5.2	**Responsibilities of Compounding Personnel**
5.2-1	What training is required for compounding CSPs?
5.2-2	What are the key competencies that compounders must demonstrate?
5.3	**Documenting Competence**
5.3-1	What competence information has to be documented?
5.3-2	How often should training occur?
5.3-3	Is there a set number of training hours required?
5.3-4	Do pharmacists who only check—but don't compound—CSPs have to document competency?
5.3-5	I am at a small hospital and the only pharmacist. How can I document my competency?
5.4	**Hazard Communication Plan**
5.4-1	What is a hazard communication plan?
5.4-2	Is a hazardous chemical the same thing as a hazardous drug?
5.4-3	Where can I find safety data sheets?
5.4-4	Do all drugs require an SDS?
5.4-5	Whose responsibility is it to develop a hazard communication plan?

SECTION 6: POLICIES AND PROCEDURES

6.1	What type of policies should I have?
6.2	Are SOPs and policies the same thing?
6.3	Do the policies have to be written?
6.4	Who, and at what frequency, needs to review policies?
6.5	How long do I have to keep old policies?

LIST OF QUESTIONS (continued)

SECTION 7: GARB AND HAND HYGIENE

7.1	**General Information**
7.1-1	What does <797> require for garb?
7.1-2	What is the purpose of garb?
7.1-3	Is there a difference between garb and PPE?
7.1-4	Is different garb required for hazardous and nonhazardous CSPs?
7.1-5	Is additional garb required for personnel who are compounding from powders?
7.1-6	Do I need to wear garb if the hood I work in is a glove box?
7.1-7	What does *donning* and *doffing* mean?
7.1-8	Does the pharmacist who is only checking items need to garb?
7.1-9	Can garb be reused?
7.1-10	The pharmacists and technicians who work in our operating room (OR) satellite wear "OR greens." Is this sufficient garb?
7.2	**Hand Hygiene**
7.2-1	What does *hand hygiene* mean?
7.2-2	Can alcohol-based hand gel be used instead of soap and water?
7.2-3	How long should our policy say to wash hands?
7.2-4	Are regular paper towels OK to use?
7.3	**Gloves**
7.3-1	When gloves are mentioned in <797>, what kind of gloves does that mean?
7.3-2	Is it OK to wash gloves between compounds?
7.3-3	When are sterile gloves required?
7.3-4	We use glove boxes to put on gloves outside of the glove box. Is this correct?
7.3-5	Are sterile gloves required when working in a compounding isolator?
7.3-6	How often do compounding isolator gloves need to be changed?
7.3-7	Do chemo gloves have to meet a particular standard?
7.3-8	How do I know if a glove is chemo-rated?
7.3-9	Is it OK for chemo gloves to be tested per ASTM D6978 and laboratory chemical tested per ASTM F739?
7.4	**Gowns**
7.4-1	Do gowns have to be sterile?
7.4-2	What is the difference between gowns we use for non-HDs and those used for chemo?
7.4-3	Can I hang my gown in the anteroom for use later in the day?
7.4-4	Are washable gowns OK to use?
7.4-5	Do I need to wear a regular gown under my chemo gown?
7.5	**Hair Covers**
7.5-1	What is the difference between head and beard covers used for chemo and those used for nonhazardous CSPs?
7.5-2	One of our employees is completely bald. Does he need to wear a hair cover?
7.5-3	If personnel wear a head cover for religious or other reasons, is an additional hair cover necessary?
7.5-4	Do earrings have to be removed, or can they just be covered by the hair cover?

LIST OF QUESTIONS (continued)

7.6	Masks
7.6-1	Do I have to wear a surgical mask when compounding?
7.6-2	Is a mask the same thing as a respirator?
7.6-3	Is a face shield a mask?
7.7	Sleeves
7.7-1	Are sleeve covers required?
7.8	Shoe Covers
7.8-1	What is the difference between shoe covers used for chemo and those used for non-HDs?
7.8-2	Can I use dedicated cleanroom shoes instead of shoe covers?
7.9	Eye Protection
7.9-1	What does *eye protection* mean?
7.9-2	I wear prescription eyeglasses. Does this qualify as eye protection?
7.9-3	I wear a face shield to protect my contact lenses from drying out. Is this proper eye protection?
7.9-4	Do I need eye protection when I'm cleaning up a spill?
7.10	Respiratory Protection
7.10-1	What does *respiratory protection* mean?
7.10-2	What does an N95 respirator protect against?
7.10-3	Are there respirators that are better protection than N95?
7.10-4	Do surgical masks provide adequate respiratory protection?
7.10-5	Because the biological safety cabinet (BSC) and CACI provide respiratory protection, do I need to wear a regular mask for any HD compounding?
7.10-6	Do I need respiratory protection when I'm cleaning up a spill?
7.11	Garbing Procedures
7.11-1	What garb components are garbed first?
7.11-2	We put on hair covers, shoe covers, and masks before entering the clean side of the anteroom. In what order should these be donned?
7.11-3	What is the proper order of donning garb for compounding CSPs in a cleanroom suite (positive pressure anteroom with sink on the clean side of the anteroom and positive pressure buffer room)?
7.11-4	What is the proper order of donning garb for compounding CSPs in an SCA with a sink inside the room but outside the perimeter around the PEC?
7.11-5	My facility design is different from the two examples above. Do I need to use only the order listed?
7.11-6	Is additional garb required for personnel who are compounding from powders?

SECTION 8: IMMEDIATE USE AND PREPARATION FOR ADMINISTRATION

8.1	What is considered *immediate use*?
8.2	What is considered *administration*?
8.3	What is considered *preparation for administration*?
8.4	Can nurses mix compounded sterile preparations (CSPs) for immediate use?
8.5	Can staff other than nurses mix CSPs for immediate use?
8.6	Can pharmacy personnel mix CSPs for immediate use?
8.7	Is reconstitution of an antibiotic vial considered immediate use or preparation for administration?
8.8	Is there any difference between the previous definition of immediate use and the definition in the revised <797>?

LIST OF QUESTIONS (continued)

8.9	What's the difference between using three sterile containers and using three different sterile products?
8.10	How long after someone mixes an immediate-use IV does it have to be used?
8.11	The previous version of <797> required that an immediate-use IV was hung within 1 hour of preparation. The revision says 4 hours. Which is correct?
8.12	I thought immediate use meant to use it right away. Do we have to use a 4-hour beyond-use date for these IVs?
8.13	Can a Banana Bag be mixed under the immediate-use definition?
8.14	Is it OK to let the night nursing supervisors enter the pharmacy to use the IV hood?
8.15	Our pharmacy is not open 24 hours. The nurses in ICU occasionally need to mix a sodium bicarbonate IV stat. Is this OK using the immediate-use definition?
8.16	When anesthesia staff prepare syringes for cases, is this the immediate-use provision?
8.17	Do nurses and anesthesia personnel need to complete the same competency to mix IVs that pharmacists and pharmacy techs need to do?
8.18	Do personnel who prepare only immediate-use IVs need to complete a media fill and gloved fingertip and thumb test?
8.19	Our pre-op area spikes a case of liters of Lactated Ringers for the following morning use. Is this OK under the immediate-use provision?
8.20	One of our physicians is a dermatologist. Her staff prepares buffered lidocaine syringes for the day's use. Is this OK under the immediate-use provision?
8.21	One of our physician's offices has an allergy clinic. His staff mixes allergen extracts for patient use. Is this OK under the immediate-use provision?

SECTION 9: PERSONNEL TRAINING AND COMPETENCE DOCUMENTATION

9.1	**Initial Training**
9.1-1	What initial training is required to mix compounded sterile preparations (CSPs)?
9.1-2	What are the core competencies that a compounder must demonstrate?
9.1-3	Should I hire only personnel with prior IV room experience?
9.1-4	If people have documented training from other hospitals, do I need to train them?
9.1-5	What resources are available for training materials?
9.1-6	If a pharmacist has BPS board certification, do they need additional training?
9.1-7	If a technician has technician certification, do they need additional training?
9.1-8	If a technician has both a CPhT and the additional sterile compounding certification, do they need additional training?
9.1-9	Our clerkship students are trained by the college prior to coming to hospital sites. Do they need additional training?
9.1-10	Who has to oversee the training and check off new personnel?
9.1-11	Can a technician be the person who OKs a staff member's training, or does it have to be a pharmacist?
9.1-12	Does training need to be documented?
9.1-13	Does training documentation have to be written?
9.1-14	Do people who aren't compounding need training if they enter the IV room?
9.1-15	If pharmacists just check IVs but don't compound, do they need training?
9.1-16	I'm the only pharmacist. Who has to train me?

LIST OF QUESTIONS (continued)

9.2	**Hand Hygiene**
9.2-1	Is hand hygiene the same thing as hand washing?
9.2-2	Where can I find a comprehensive description of hand hygiene?
9.2-3	Is soap and water OK to use for hand hygiene?
9.2-4	How often does a compounder need to demonstrate proper hand hygiene?
9.2-5	Do people who are just checking IVs need to show competence in hand hygiene?
9.3	**Garbing**
9.3-1	How often does a compounder need to demonstrate proper garbing?
9.3-2	Do people who are just checking IVs need to demonstrate proper garbing procedures?
9.4	**Gloved Fingertip and Thumb Test**
9.4-1	What is the purpose of the gloved fingertip and thumb test?
9.4-2	What type of media is used for a gloved fingertip and thumb test?
9.4-3	What is the proper procedure for doing a gloved fingertip and thumb test?
9.4-4	Where are the samples kept?
9.4-5	How are the samples incubated?
9.4-6	How and where is the initial gloved fingertip and thumb test done?
9.4-7	Can a person garb once and use three sets of plates at one time for the initial gloved fingertip and thumb test?
9.4-8	Do the three separate garbing sessions need to be done on the same day?
9.4-9	How and where is the requalification gloved fingertip and thumb test done?
9.4-10	We use a compounding aseptic isolator (CAI). Does the gloved fingertip and thumb test need to be done inside the CAI?
9.4-11	How often is the requalification gloved fingertip and thumb test required?
9.4-12	Are three sets of media plates required for the requalification gloved fingertip and thumb test?
9.4-13	If someone passes two of the initial three gloved fingertip and thumb tests, do they have to repeat all three or just one?
9.4-14	Is the training gloved fingertip and thumb test different from the one for retraining?
9.4-15	What does the *action level* mean?
9.4-16	Do the action level numbers apply to one hand or both hands?
9.4-17	Do you need to sample both hands?
9.4-18	Can one plate be used for both hands?
9.4-19	What is the action level for the initial gloved fingertip and thumb test?
9.4-20	What is the action level for the requalification gloved fingertip and thumb test?
9.4-21	Why must I have no growth on a gloved fingertip and thumb test when I'm learning, but when I'm really mixing IVs for patients, I can have some growth?
9.4-22	If someone exceeds the action level, can they compound?
9.4-23	Do nurses who only mix immediate-use CSPs need to do a gloved fingertip and thumb test?
9.4-24	Do the nuclear medicine technologists need to do a gloved fingertip and thumb test?
9.5	**Aseptic Technique**
9.5-1	What is the definition of *aseptic technique*?
9.5-2	Is there a USP chapter about aseptic technique?
9.5-3	Does ASHP have any resources to teach aseptic technique?

LIST OF QUESTIONS (continued)

9.5-4	Is the aseptic technique nurses learn or the technique used in the operating room (OR) the same thing as the aseptic technique we need to use when compounding?
9.5-5	What test is used to demonstrate competence in aseptic technique?
9.6	**Media Fill Test**
9.6-1	What is the purpose of the media fill test?
9.6-2	How often does a media fill test have to be done?
9.6-3	How do I design a media fill test?
9.6-4	Can I use a commercially available kit for a media fill test?
9.6-5	What kind of media and devices are used for a media fill test?
9.6-6	We use a CAI. Do we still need to do a media fill test?
9.6-7	Does everyone on staff need to do the same media fill test?
9.6-8	What is the proper procedure for doing a media fill test?
9.6-9	If I mix nonsterile-to-sterile preparations, can I use purchased soybean-casein digest media?
9.6-10	Can I start with nonsterile media and mix it myself?
9.6-11	Is there specific information I need to keep concerning the media used?
9.6-12	Do I need an incubator?
9.6-13	Can I use a mannitol warmer to incubate the media fill tests?
9.6-14	At what temperature and for how long do the media fill tests need to be incubated?
9.6-15	Is there an action level for media fill tests?
9.6-16	Where is the initial media fill test done?
9.6-17	Where is the requalification media fill test done?
9.6-18	What should be documented?
9.6-19	Do nurses who only mix immediate-use CSPs need to do a media fill test?
9.6-20	Do the nuclear medicine technologists need to do a media fill test?
9.7	**Requalification**
9.7-1	How often does retraining need to occur?
9.7-2	If someone has been on leave, or has not compounded for a while, do they need to demonstrate competence before they can compound?
9.7-3	Do I need to document the requalification?
9.7-4	Who needs to keep the records for training? Pharmacy? Human Resources? The individual?

SECTION 10: STERILE PRODUCTS AND SUPPLIES

10.1	**General Information**
10.1-1	What is the difference between the terms *products* and *preparations*?
10.1-2	What are conventionally manufactured products?
10.1-3	Does <797> deal with manufactured products? I thought it was only about compounded sterile preparations.
10.1-4	What are considered components of a CSP?
10.2	**Use of Nonsterile Starting Components**
10.2-1	What is an API?
10.2-2	Do all components need to be marked *USP* or *NF*?
10.2-3	Why do I have to use API that's from an FDA-registered supplier?

LIST OF QUESTIONS (continued)

10.2-4	I need to use an excipient that doesn't have a *USP* or *NF* monograph. Where do I get it?
10.2-5	How do I know the quality of the component?
10.2-6	Is water a component?
10.2-7	I have some chemicals marked ACS. Are they OK to use?
10.2-8	I have a shelf full of old chemicals. Many are marked *USP* or *NF*. Are they OK to use?
10.2-9	If I received a chemical without an expiration date, do I need to assign a date?
10.2-10	Can I start the 1-year expiry from the date I open the jar?
10.2-11	The alum we use has a manufacturer's expiration date. Do I need to discard it after 1 year?

SECTION 11: FACILITY DESIGN, ENGINEERING CONTROLS, AND EQUIPMENT

11.1	**General Facility Design Information**
11.1-1	What are the minimum facility requirements for compounding sterile preparations?
11.1-2	Are there different minimum facility requirements for compounding hazardous sterile preparations?
11.1-3	What engineering controls are required by <797>?
11.1-4	Is an engineering control and a PEC the same thing?
11.1-5	What does *classified* mean?
11.1-6	Does the sterile compounding area need to be a separate room?
11.1-7	Can noncompounding activities occur in the compounding area?
11.1-8	Is it OK to use part of the intravenous (IV) room for office-related space, like order entry and processing?
11.1-9	Is there a restriction concerning who can enter the IV room?
11.1-10	How much space is necessary for compounding?
11.1-11	Can I use plastic curtains or drapes to define the compounding area?
11.1-12	Does the hood need to be on emergency power?
11.1-13	Can I use the same compounding room for both nonhazardous and hazardous sterile compounding?
11.1-14	Do I need a separate room for receiving sterile products?
11.1-15	What type of sink do I need, and where should it be placed?
11.1-16	Should the sink be next to the hood?
11.1-17	Why does a sink need to be at least 1 meter away from the hood?
11.1-18	Should the garb storage be adjacent to the sink?
11.1-19	Are there any temperature or humidity requirements for the sterile compounding area?
11.1-20	If the humidity is low, should I put in a humidifier?
11.1-21	What are the minimum air changes per hour required by <797>?
11.1-22	Can I depend on any type of PEC to be able to contribute 15 ACPH?
11.1-23	Because <797> lists minimum number of ACPH, is there any need to use a higher number?
11.1-24	How many ACPH are required for an SCA?
11.1-25	Where should the gauges be for the temperature, humidity, and pressure?
11.1-26	What kind of finishes do I need to use for floors, walls, and ceilings?
11.1-27	What documents should my certifier reference on certification reports?
11.2	**Storage Areas**
11.2-1	I have heard that cardboard isn't allowed in the compounding area. Is that true?
11.2-2	Can shipping boxes be taken into the compounding area?

LIST OF QUESTIONS (continued)

11.2-3	IV bags and other supplies used for compounding come in cardboard boxes. What is the best way to store these?
11.2-4	Do storage rooms require a specific ACPH?
11.2-5	Is it OK to store supplies on the floor?
11.3	**Primary Engineering Controls**
11.3-1	What should I look for when buying a hood?
11.3-2	How often do hoods for sterile compounding have to be certified?
11.3-3	Is there an industry guidance for testing/certification of a hood?
11.3-4	Is it OK to turn off the hood when we aren't using it?
11.3-5	Can I use the same device for both nonhazardous and chemo sterile compounding?
11.3-6	Is a robot a PEC?
11.3-7	How many people can work in one hood?
11.3-8	Does the pressure need to be documented every day for the space in the CAI?
11.3-9	Are CAIs Category 1 or Category 2 CSPs?
11.3-10	Does a CAI need to be in a cleanroom suite?
11.3-11	We have a system that includes a camera inside the hood. Is this OK?
11.3-12	We have a system that includes a scale inside the hood. Is this OK?
11.3-13	We have a system that includes a touchscreen monitor inside the hood. Is this OK?
11.4	**Secondary Engineering Control—General Information**
11.4-1	What is a secondary engineering control (SEC)?
11.4-2	Are modular rooms OK to have?
11.4-3	What kind of things do I need to be sure our architects, facility department, and contractor need to consider when designing our IV room?
11.4-4	Do all surfaces have to be stainless steel?
11.4-5	Is every sterile compounding room an SEC?
11.4-6	Is an SEC positive or negative pressure, or can it be neutral pressure?
11.4-7	Is a chemo room an SEC?
11.4-8	How big should an SEC be?
11.4-9	Is it OK to use the SEC for order entry if it's related to sterile compounding?
11.4-10	Can the SEC be used to store drugs, IV solutions, and supplies?
11.4-11	Can I put shelving in my sterile compounding area?
11.4-12	Can I put a refrigerator in my sterile compounding area?
11.4-13	Can I put a printer in my sterile compounding area?
11.4-14	How do I calculate room air change rates?
11.4-15	Do the monitors for temperature, humidity, and pressure have to be inside the IV room?
11.4-16	What is the distinction between the dirty and clean side of an SEC?
11.5	**Anterooms**
11.5-1	What is an anteroom?
11.5-2	What are the physical requirements for an anteroom?
11.5-3	Does every sterile compounding room need an anteroom?
11.5-4	Is an anteroom positive or negative pressure, or can it be neutral pressure?

LIST OF QUESTIONS (continued)

11.5-5	Because our chemo room is negative pressure, does the anteroom for that need to be negative pressure?
11.5-6	Is more than one anteroom required if we have a positive and a negative buffer room?
11.5-7	How big should an anteroom be?
11.5-8	Is there a minimum square footage requirement?
11.5-9	Is there a minimum square footage requirement based on the number of people in the room?
11.5-10	Is it OK to use the anteroom for order entry if it's related to sterile compounding?
11.5-11	Can the anteroom have a pneumatic tube?
11.5-12	Can the anteroom be used to store drugs, IV solutions, and supplies?
11.5-13	Can the anteroom have shelves?
11.5-14	What is the distinction between the dirty and clean side of an anteroom?
11.5-15	What is the line of demarcation in the anteroom?
11.5-16	What is the distinction between a wet and dry anteroom?
11.5-17	Can the anteroom have a sink?
11.5-18	Does the anteroom have to have a sink?
11.5-19	My SCA is ISO 7. Does it need an anteroom?
11.5-20	If I put a CAI in the anteroom, is that considered a cleanroom suite?
11.5-21	What kind of finishes should be used for the floor, walls, and ceiling of an anteroom?
11.5-22	Is it OK to separate the sides of an anteroom by putting tape on the floor?
11.6	**Presterilization Area for Weighing Powders**
11.6-1	Where should powders be weighed for preparation of sterile CSPs?
11.6-2	Do I need a separate area for weighing powders if I never mix CSPs from nonsterile ingredients?
11.7	**Cleanroom Suites**
11.7-1	What are the minimum room requirements for a cleanroom suite?
11.7-2	What does a cleanroom suite have that an SCA doesn't have?
11.7-3	I have a combined ante/buffer room. Is this a cleanroom suite?
11.7-4	What is the ISO requirement for a cleanroom suite?
11.7-5	Are ceiling HEPA filters required?
11.7-6	I have HEPA filters in the ceiling and the air returns about a foot down from the ceiling. Is this OK?
11.7-7	Does a cleanroom suite require an isolator?
11.7-8	I have a combined anteroom/buffer room that is ISO 7. I heard this is no longer allowed in new <797>. Is this true?
11.7-9	Where does the sink need to be placed in a cleanroom suite?
11.7-10	Are there separate requirements for a cleanroom suite used for chemo?
11.7-11	Can the air conditioning be turned off in the cleanroom suite when it's not in use?
11.7-12	Can the number of air changes per hour be lowered when the cleanroom suite is not in use?
11.7-13	Are portable HEPA filters OK to use?
11.7-14	How many people can work in a cleanroom suite?
11.8	**Segregated Compounding Areas for Nonhazardous CSPs**
11.8-1	What are the minimum room requirements for an SCA?
11.8-2	What can be mixed in an SCA?
11.8-3	Can all CSPs be mixed in an SCA?

LIST OF QUESTIONS (continued)

11.8-4	What does a cleanroom suite have that an SCA doesn't have?
11.8-5	What is the purpose of a perimeter around the hood?
11.8-6	Where does the sink need to be placed in an SCA?
11.8-7	Are there separate requirements for an SCA used for chemo?
11.8-8	What is the ISO requirement for an SCA?
11.9	**Containment Segregated Compounding Areas for Hazardous CSPs**
11.9-1	What are the minimum room requirements for a C-SCA?
11.9-2	Can I use a C-SCA for mixing all CSPs—both hazardous and not?
11.9-3	What does a cleanroom suite have that a C-SCA doesn't have?
11.9-4	Where does the sink need to be placed in a C-SCA?
11.9-5	What is the ISO requirement for a C-SCA?
11.10	**Pass-Through Chambers**
11.10-1	What is a pass-through?
11.10-2	What components make a pass-through cleanroom-compliant?
11.10-3	How big can a pass-through chamber be?
11.10-4	Can a pass-through go from unclassified space into a cleanroom?
11.10-5	What testing is needed for a pass-through chamber?
11.10-6	How can I tell if the pass-through is contributing to problems in the IV room?
11.10-7	We have a window that slides open between the anteroom and buffer room. Is this a pass-through chamber?
11.10-8	Is a window OK in the pass-through chamber?
11.10-9	Does the pass-through chamber need to be HEPA-filtered?
11.10-10	I have a HEPA-filtered pass-through. Can I turn off the HEPA filter when it's not in use?
11.10-11	Do HEPA-filtered pass-throughs need to be ISO classified?
11.10-12	How big are pass-through chambers?
11.10-13	Is it OK to pass supplies through a pass-through?
11.10-14	Our pass-through isn't interlocked, but we only allow opening one side at a time. Is this OK?
11.10-15	We have a pass-through that is interlocked, but I can feel air moving in from the other room. Is this OK?
11.10-16	Is a cart-sized pass-through OK to have?
11.10-17	Is a pass-through refrigerator OK to have?
11.11	**Refrigerator and Freezer Placement**
11.11-1	Is it OK to have refrigerators or freezers in a sterile compounding area?
11.11-2	What type of refrigerator is required?
11.11-3	What does a "low wall return" for a refrigerator mean?
11.11-4	Is a pass-through refrigerator OK to have?
11.12	**Other Compounding Area Equipment**
11.12-1	What other kind of equipment is used for sterile compounding?
11.12-2	How do I know that mechanical equipment is OK to use?
11.12-3	How can I be sure the equipment is USP-compliant?
11.12-4	Can I have a telephone in the sterile compounding area?
11.12-5	Can I have a printer in the sterile compounding area?
11.12-6	We use a system that has a computer tablet in the hood. Is this OK?

LIST OF QUESTIONS (continued)

11.12-7	Is it OK to have a warmer in the sterile compounding area?
11.12-8	Is it OK to have an incubator in the sterile compounding area?
11.12-9	Is there a requirement to calibrate the equipment?
11.13	**Compounding Immediate-Use CSPs in Ambient Air**
11.13-1	What does *ambient air* mean?
11.13-2	Why is it OK to mix CSPs outside of an IV room?
11.13-3	Is the OR considered ambient air?
11.13-4	What minimum requirements should an area used for immediate-use preparations have?
11.13-5	If IVs are mixed in ambient air, do those areas need to be included in environmental monitoring?
11.13-6	Is a doctor's office considered ambient air?
11.14	**Allergenic Extracts Compounding Area**
11.14-1	Do allergen extracts have to be prepared in an IV room?
11.14-2	Do allergen extracts have to be prepared in an SCA?
11.14-3	The allergists at our health system want to comply with <797>. What choices do they have for facility design?
11.14-4	What is an AECA?
11.14-5	If a pharmacy prepares allergen extracts, does it need to be done in a regular IV room or is an AECA required?
11.14-6	Does an AECA require a hood?
11.14-7	When is it OK to use an AECA?
11.14-8	Can only doctor's offices have an AECA?
11.15	**Segregated Radiopharmaceutical Processing Area**
11.15-1	Can radiopharmaceuticals be mixed in the regular pharmacy IV room?
11.15-2	Can radiopharmaceuticals be mixed in the laboratory's BSC?
11.15-3	Does the nuclear medicine department need an IV room?
11.15-4	Does the nuclear medicine department need a hood?
11.15-5	What is an SRPA?
11.15-6	Does my nuclear medicine department require an SRPA?

SECTION 12: DAILY NONVIABLE MONITORING

12.1	What monitoring is required to be done daily?
12.2	What's the difference between nonviable and viable monitoring?
12.3	What's the difference between certification and monitoring?
12.4	What monitoring is the certifier required to do?
12.5	Our certifier also does the viable testing. Is this OK?
12.6	What should the temperature of the sterile compounding areas be?
12.7	What do I need to do if it's too cold in the sterile compounding area?
12.8	What do I need to do if it's too warm in the sterile compounding area?
12.9	Do I need to monitor the temperature of storage areas outside the intravenous (IV) room?
12.10	What should the humidity be in the sterile compounding area?
12.11	What should I do if the humidity is too low?

LIST OF QUESTIONS (continued)

12.12	My facilities department says the humidity has to be at least 20%. They want to add a humidifier. Is that OK?
12.13	What should I do if the humidity is too high?
12.14	Can we use a dehumidifier to correct humidity that is too high?
12.15	What should I do if the pressure in my anteroom or positive pressure buffer room is too positive?
12.16	What should I do if the pressure in my negative pressure buffer room or C-SCA is too negative?
12.17	If temperature, humidity, or pressure is out of range, do I have to report this to someone?
12.18	How often does our automated compounding device (ACD) need to be tested?
12.19	How often does our repeater pump need to be tested?

SECTION 13: CERTIFICATION OF ENGINEERING CONTROLS

13.1	What does *certification* mean? How is it different from the monitoring I have to do every day?
13.2	What qualifications does a certifier need?
13.3	What is CETA?
13.4	What are CETA CAGs?
13.5	What should my certification report include?
13.6	What does *dynamic conditions* mean?
13.7	Can I compound while the certifier is working in the room?
13.8	Does the certifier need access to the ceiling above the intravenous (IV) room?
13.9	Is there a way to test the ceiling HEPA filters without crawling in the ceiling?
13.10	My hood failed certification. Can I use it?
13.11	My room failed certification. Can I use it?
13.12	We use an ACD. Should we take it out of the hood when the certifier tests the hood?
13.13	We use a repeater pump. Should we take it out of the hood when the certifier tests the hood?
13.14	We use an IV software system that has equipment in the hood. Should we take it out of the hood when the certifier tests the hood?
13.15	Should the certifier do our environmental monitoring?
13.16	If the power goes off in our hood or room, does it need to be recertified before we can use it again?
13.17	Our certifier says our chemo room is "too negative" and that it's OK now but won't be in the future. Is this correct?
13.18	Do we have to get our hoods and rooms certified before we use them?
13.19	When does a hood need to be certified?
13.20	When does a room need to be certified?
13.21	Can my facilities department check my hood?
13.22	We have a powder hood in our negative pressure storage room. Does it need to be retested every 6 months or every year?

SECTION 14: COMPOUNDING

14.1	**General Information**
14.1-1	How many people are allowed in the sterile compounding area?
14.1-2	Can students compound sterile preparations? If not, how can they learn?
14.1-3	Are cellphones allowed in the sterile compounding areas?
14.1-4	Is it OK to play music in the sterile compounding area?

LIST OF QUESTIONS (continued)

14.1-5	Is mixing immediate-use compounded sterile preparations (CSPs) considered compounding?
14.1-6	What special policies and procedures are needed for compounding intrathecal or epidural CSPs?
14.1-7	Are vial tops sterile when they come from the manufacturer?
14.1-8	Are there some drugs that I should not compound?
14.1-9	Is the bulk list the same for pharmacies and for outsourcing facilities?
14.1-10	Is prepackaging medications into syringe containers considered compounding?
14.1-11	Does ASHP have guidelines dealing with sterile compounding?
14.1-12	Are premixed solutions that I can buy from manufacturers considered compounded?
14.1-13	Are premixed solutions that I can buy from an outsourcing facility considered compounded?
14.1-14	Is reconstituting a system like an ADD-Vantage™, MINI-BAG Plus, VIAL-MATE, or addEASE® considered compounding?
14.1-15	If I crush tablets or open capsules to make a CSP, is that active pharmaceutical ingredient (API)?
14.1-16	Is there an algorithm I can use to determine if it's appropriate to compound?
14.2	**Nonsterile-to-Sterile Compounding**
14.2-1	How do I know if an ingredient is nonsterile?
14.2-2	Do I need a Certificate of Analysis for every ingredient in a compound?
14.2-3	How are CSPs that start with nonsterile components sterilized?
14.2-4	What is the difference between terminal sterilization and filtration?
14.2-5	What is a bubble point test?
14.2-6	Do containers need to be sterile?
14.2-7	Is it OK to use an amber dropper bottle for sterile CSPs?
14.2-8	If I batch 50 cefazolin syringes, do I need to do sterility tests?
14.2-9	Are there additional requirements when working with blood components?
14.2-10	Are there additional requirements when working with albumin, IVIG, vaccines, or other biologics?
14.2-11	Are there additional requirements when working with radiopharmaceuticals like UltraTag™?
14.3	**Master Formulation Records**
14.3-1	What is a master formulation record?
14.3-2	When is an MFR needed?
14.3-3	What needs to be recorded in an MFR?
14.3-4	Is there a template form I can use to create an MFR?
14.3-5	We have a file with recipes for compounds. Is this the same as an MFR?
14.3-6	Where are sources of compounds available?
14.3-7	If I make two different strengths of a CSP, do I need one or two MFRs?
14.3-8	Do I need to make an MFR for a one-time order or prescription?
14.3-9	Can I combine the MFR with a compounding record?
14.3-10	Is it OK to double or halve the listing on the MFR?
14.3-11	Do the MFRs have to be printed out?
14.3-12	What happens if a change has to be made in an MFR?
14.3-13	When changes are necessary, who can make them?
14.3-14	Do I need an MFR for every antibiotic CSP I make?
14.3-15	Does the MFR need to be in a specific format?

LIST OF QUESTIONS (continued)

14.4	**Compounding Records**
14.4-1	What is a compounding record?
14.4-2	When is a CR needed?
14.4-3	What needs to be recorded in a CR?
14.4-4	I've always recorded the information above for batches, but not for "one offs"—a single bag or two for one patient for a specific order. Do I need a CR for those?
14.4-5	Do I have to record manufacturer's lot numbers for every CSP?
14.4-6	Is there a template form I can use to create a CR?
14.4-7	Do the CRs have to be printed out?
14.5	**Allergenic Extracts**
14.5-1	How are allergenic extracts compounded?
14.6	**Radiopharmaceuticals**
14.6-1	How are radiopharmaceuticals compounded?
14.6-2	Is there a difference between what an outside nuclear pharmacy compounds and what is compounded in the hospital's nuclear medicine department?

SECTION 15: BEYOND-USE DATES

15.1	**General Beyond-Use Date Information**
15.1-1	Is a beyond-use date the same thing as an expiration date?
15.1-2	What's the difference among an expiration date, beyond-use day, in-use time, and infusion time?
15.1-3	What factors go into the determination of a BUD?
15.1-4	We have a cleanroom suite and mix CSPs from commercially available sterile products. What is the maximum BUD we can use?
15.1-5	We make all CSPs in a SCA. What is the maximum BUD we can use?
15.1-6	We make all our chemos in a containment segregated compounding area (C-SCA). What is the maximum BUD we can use?
15.1-7	We have a cleanroom suite and occasionally mix CSPs from nonsterile starting ingredients. What is the maximum BUD we can use?
15.1-8	Can we mix CSPs from nonsterile ingredients in an SCA?
15.1-9	We filter some CSPs mixed from nonsterile ingredients. Do we use the information about aseptically prepared or terminally sterilized CSPs listed in <797>?
15.1-10	What is a USP monograph?
15.1-11	Where can I find a USP monograph?
15.1-12	If we use a USP monograph, can we use the BUD listed in the monograph?
15.1-13	Can I use a USP monograph and extend the BUD beyond what's listed in the monograph?
15.1-14	Can I use BUDs longer than those listed in <797> if I have peer-reviewed information that states a longer BUD?
15.1-15	If a drug's stability information is less than the BUD in <797>, can I still use the <797> BUD?
15.1-16	What are the required temperature ranges for room temperature, refrigerated, and frozen CSPs?
15.1-17	Are temperatures listed in <797> in Celsius or Fahrenheit?
15.1-18	Does the BUD include the time the drug is infused?
15.1-19	How do I know how long a CSP will be infused?
15.1-20	Does the term *used* in <797> include the infusion time?
15.1-21	How do I know to use the aseptic processing BUDs or the terminal sterilization BUDs?

LIST OF QUESTIONS (continued)

15.1-22	Is a summary of the maximum BUD times available?
15.1-23	We reconstitute and freeze some antibiotic syringes. Can I keep them for 45 days, then move them to the refrigerator for another 10 days?
15.1-24	We reconstitute and refrigerate some antibiotic syringes and give them a 10 day BUD. If we take them out of the refrigerator on day 4, what is the room temperature BUD?
15.1-25	We warm some solutions (either before use or after compounding). What is the BUD for solutions placed in warmers?
15.1-26	Can I extend the BUDs beyond those listed in <797>?
15.1-27	I have published studies that have BUDs of 1 or 2 years. Can I use them?
15.1-28	I have published studies that show 100% of the compound remaining on day 30. Can I extrapolate that information to use a longer BUD?
15.1-29	Is it always OK to use the default dates listed in <797>?
15.1-30	If I make a CSP today, does the time for the BUD start today or tomorrow?
15.1-31	Do BUDs for intrathecal or epidural CSPs need to be less than those defaults listed in <797>?
15.1-32	Pharmacy references often have stability information that is longer than the BUDs allowed in <797>. Can I use the references?
15.1-33	My state has the old BUDs in regulations. Do I follow them or new <797> information?
15.1-34	Do the BUDs in <797> apply to compounds made for animals?
15.1-35	Does the BUD differ based on the category of compound (low, medium, or high risk)?
15.2	**Active Pharmaceutical Ingredients and Other Components**
15.2-1	What is the BUD of opened jars of components?
15.2-2	What should I do with old bottles of chemicals and other components?
15.2-3	Can the container used for the package of a CSP affect the stability?
15.3	**Vial/Bag Systems**
15.3-1	What is the BUD of products like ADD-Vantage™, MiniBag Plus, VIAL-MATE, addEASE® and similar systems?
15.4	**Vials and Other Dosage Forms**
15.4-1	Do BUDs apply to manufactured products, or only compounded preparations?
15.4-2	What is the BUD of a single-dose ampule?
15.4-3	What's the BUD of a single-dose vial?
15.4-4	Is a manufactured IV bag (like a saline bag used for reconstituting antibiotics) a single-dose or a multiple-dose container?
15.4-5	Once an IV is spiked, what is the BUD?
15.4-6	Is the BUD of a manufactured solution different from a compounded CSP?
15.4-7	What's the BUD of an IV made during a code?
15.4-8	When I go in the operating room (OR) prep room on evenings, I see several cases of IV solutions spiked and hanging. The OR says this is standard practice and there is no BUD. Is this correct?
15.4-9	Is a manufactured irrigation bottle a single-dose or a multiple-dose container?
15.4-10	What is the BUD of a multiple-dose vial?
15.4-11	Once punctured, should a multiple-dose vial be refrigerated or kept in the hood?
15.4-12	If I am going to save a multiple-dose vial for future use, do I need to date it with the open date or the end date?
15.4-13	If a multiple-dose vial is missing the cap, does that affect the BUD?
15.4-14	What is the BUD of a pharmacy bulk package (PBP)?

LIST OF QUESTIONS (continued)

15.4-15	If a PBP is labeled with a manufacturer's in-use time of 4 hours, can I still use it for 12 hours since I opened it under the hood?
15.5	**Compounded Stock Bags**
15.5-1	We mix an electrolyte bag to use in neonatal TPNs. How long is the bag good for?
15.5-2	Our 503B outsourcing facility mixes stock bags for us. Do they have a different BUD than if I mixed them myself?

SECTION 16: DISPENSING AND PACKAGING

16.1	What are some key issues to confirm when dispensing a compounded sterile preparation?
16.2	What has to be on the label of a compounded sterile preparation?
16.3	What's the difference between the label and the labeling?
16.4	Why would there be a different spot to put a label on a CSP?
16.5	Does a CSP label have to include the fact that it is compounded?
16.6	Does the technician who mixed the CSP and the pharmacist who checked the CSP need to initial the label?
16.7	Are there requirements for the packaging that must be used for CSPs that are mailed or shipped?
16.8	Are temperature monitors required for CSPs that are shipped?

SECTION 17: CLEANING AND DISINFECTING

17.1	**General Information**
17.1-1	What is the difference between deactivating, decontaminating, cleaning, and disinfecting?
17.1-2	<800> mentions decontaminating, but <797> doesn't. Why? Do I still need to decontaminate my chemo areas?
17.1-3	<797> mentions use of sporicidals. Why?
17.1-4	Which is done first: cleaning or disinfecting?
17.1-5	Do I need to wear garb when cleaning?
17.1-6	What does *dwell time* mean?
17.1-7	We always clean with sterile alcohol. Is that enough?
17.1-8	Is alcohol a sanitizing agent?
17.1-9	Can an ultraviolet light be used to sanitize an area?
7.1-10	Is sterile alcohol required in <797>?
17.1-11	Should cleaning agents be rotated?
17.1-12	Are reusable mops acceptable to use?
17.1-13	What is the best way to monitor that cleaning has been done?
17.1-14	Do pharmacy personnel need to do all the cleaning of sterile compounding areas?
17.1-15	When and with what do supplies going into the sterile compounding area need to be cleaned?
17.1-16	What is a one-step cleaner? Can I use these in the intravenous (IV) room?
17.1-17	What cleaning and disinfecting needs to be done daily?
17.1-18	Does the PEC need to be cleaned and disinfected every 30 minutes?
17.1-19	What cleaning needs to be done weekly?
17.1-20	What cleaning needs to be done monthly?
17.1-21	If my IV room isn't used every day, do I still need to clean it every day?
17.1-22	Are there requirements for who can clean the IV room?

LIST OF QUESTIONS (continued)

17.1-23	How often does competency documentation for cleaning need to occur?
17.2	**Types of Cleaning Solutions**
17.2-1	How do I know what cleaning solutions to select?
17.2-2	How do I know I am using the correct dilutions of cleaning solutions?
17.2-3	Is sterile water a cleaning solution?
17.2-4	Is bleach a cleaning solution?
17.2-5	If bleach is used as a sporicidal agent, what strength should be used?
17.2-6	Once bleach is diluted, how long is it good for?
17.2-7	Are ready-to-use solutions required?
17.2-8	How should cleaning agents be applied?
17.2-9	Can any type of cloth be used for the wiper?
17.3	**Cleaning PECs and Other Compounding Equipment**
17.3-1	How often should PECs and other equipment used for compounding be cleaned?
17.3-2	What types of solutions should be used for cleaning the hoods?
17.3-3	What does *terminal cleaning* mean?
17.3-4	Who should clean the hoods?
17.3-5	How often do the hoods or other compounding surfaces need to be cleaned during compounding?
17.3-6	Do I have to clean the hoods even on days they are not used?
17.3-7	How often does an automated compounding device need to be cleaned?
17.3-8	How often does a repeater pump need to be cleaned?
17.3-9	How often does any computer equipment need to be cleaned?
17.3-10	If the power goes off, do we need to clean the hoods?
17.3-11	Do we need to clean syringes as we take them out of the packages?
17.4	**Cleaning Compounding Areas**
17.4-1	Is it OK for environmental services personnel to clean the floors while we are compounding?
17.4-2	Is alcohol sufficient to clean the compounding areas?
17.4-3	Who should clean the compounding area?
17.4-4	What is a "high-touch" area?
17.4-5	Do I have to clean the compounding area even on days it is not used?
17.4-6	How often does the office space inside the anteroom need to be cleaned?
17.4-7	How often do pass-throughs need to be cleaned?
17.4-8	How often do refrigerators in the sterile compounding area need to be cleaned?
17.4-9	Because I compound only occasionally, do I have to clean my whole pharmacy with the same frequency as the compounding area?
17.4-10	How often should I use alcohol to clean the floor?
17.5	**Cleaning Supplies Needed for Compounding**
17.5-1	When and with what should drug vials, IV bags, needles, and syringes be cleaned?

SECTION 18: ENVIRONMENTAL MONITORING

18.1	**General Information**
18.1-1	What is environmental monitoring?
18.1-2	Is environmental monitoring the same as certification?

LIST OF QUESTIONS (continued)

18.1-3	Our environmental monitoring is done by our certifier. Is that OK?	
18.1-4	Does our environmental monitoring have to be done by our certifier?	
18.1-5	What does viable monitoring do?	
18.1-6	I thought only the certifier could do air sampling. Is that correct?	
18.1-7	Do I need a detailed policy, or can I depend on what my certifier does?	
18.1-8	Do hoods and rooms need to be tested before they are used?	
18.1-9	How often does environmental monitoring need to be done?	
18.1-10	What does *commissioning* mean?	
18.1-11	What is a sampling plan?	
18.1-12	What is an action level?	
18.1-13	What is an alert level?	
18.1-14	What are highly pathogenic organisms?	
18.1-15	What is a CFU?	
18.1-16	Do I have to test for fungus if I don't make any high-risk preparations?	
18.1-17	Do I have to incubate the samples?	
18.1-18	Do I need an incubator in the pharmacy?	
18.1-19	Is a warmer OK to use to incubate the samples?	
18.1-20	Can I use the mannitol warmer to incubate the samples?	
18.1-21	Does the incubator need special controls?	
18.1-22	Can the microbiology laboratory at the hospital incubate the samples?	
18.1-23	Can an outside laboratory incubate the samples?	
18.1-24	Who should identify the growth?	
18.1-25	Can I incubate the samples in the pharmacy and send them to the laboratory for identification?	
18.1-26	Can I incubate the samples in the pharmacy and identify them myself?	
18.1-27	Does it really matter what is growing or is just the fact that there are a lot of CFUs on the plate enough information?	
18.1-28	What does *TNTC* mean on my microbiology report?	
18.2	**Active Air Sampling**	
18.2-1	What does *active air sampling* mean?	
18.2-2	What device is used to sample the air?	
18.2-3	What is measured by active air sampling?	
18.2-4	What has to be sampled?	
18.2-5	How often is active air sampling required?	
18.2-6	Do settling plates comply with <797>?	
18.2-7	Do I have to sample the air in pass-throughs?	
18.2-8	What media is used?	
18.2-9	What is the temperature required for incubators?	
18.2-10	For how long are the samples incubated?	
18.2-11	What are the action levels for active air sampling?	
18.3	**Surface Sampling**	
18.3-1	What does *surface sampling* mean?	
18.3-2	What device is used for surface sampling?	

LIST OF QUESTIONS (continued)

18.3-3	What is measured by surface sampling?
18.3-4	How often is surface sampling required?
18.3-5	What surfaces have to be sampled?
18.3-6	Do areas in the segregated compounding area (SCA) or containment segregated compounding area (C-SCA) have to be tested?
18.3-7	When is the sampling done?
18.3-8	What areas are most likely to be at risk of contamination?
18.3-9	What media is used?
18.3-10	Our laboratory doesn't stock the media listed in <797>. Can regular or blood agar plates be used?
18.3-11	What is the temperature required for incubators?
18.3-12	For how long are the samples incubated?
18.3-13	Are plates required for surface sampling or are paddles OK?
18.3-14	Is there a special type of plate to use for surface sampling?
18.3-15	Should I sample the same places each month or rotate areas?
18.3-16	What are the action levels for surface sampling?
18.4	**Reacting to Out-of-Specification Results**
18.4-1	What do I do when results are above the action level?
18.4-2	Do I need to retest when out of specification results are found?
18.4-3	There is 1 CFU of mold in the anteroom. What should I do?
18.4-4	Where are likely sources of contamination?
18.4-5	There is mold in the buffer room, but it's below the action level. What should I do?
18.4-6	My hood is OK, but my room isn't. What can I do until the room passes?
18.4-7	What results do we have to report to our state board of pharmacy?

SECTION 19: QUALITY ASSURANCE AND QUALITY CONTROL

19.1	What is the difference between quality control and quality assurance?
19.2	Does <797> define the characteristics I need to follow?
19.3	Are the components of a QA program limited to the CSPs?
19.4	What kinds of elements should we include on the report we present at the Infection Control Committee meeting?
19.5	What are considered insanitary conditions?

SECTION 20: WHAT DO I DO NOW?

20.1	I'm overwhelmed with this information. Where do I start?
20.2	Is there a template action plan I could use to start assessing the compliance at my organization?

LIST OF EXHIBITS

Exhibit 6-1. Policies Required and Recommended in USP <797>

Exhibit 9-1. Sterile Compounding Resources Available from ASHP

Exhibit 14-1. Example Master Formulation Record for CSPs

Exhibit 14-2. Example Compounding Record for CSPs

Exhibit 15-1. BUDs for Category 1 CSPs

Exhibit 15-2. BUDs for Aseptically Prepared Category 2 CSPs (Without a Sterility Test of the Final CSP) Made Only from Sterile Components

Exhibit 15-3. BUDs for Aseptically Prepared Category 2 CSPs (Without a Sterility Test of the Final CSP) Made from One or More Nonsterile Component

Exhibit 15-4. BUDs for Aseptically Prepared Category 2 CSPs That Have Passed Requirements for Sterility Testing

Exhibit 15-5. BUDs for Terminally Sterilized Category 2 CSPs Without a Sterility Test Performed or Passed

Exhibit 15-6. BUDs for Terminally Sterilized Category 2 CSPs That Have Passed Requirements for Sterility Testing

Exhibit 18-1. Action Levels for Microbial Air Sampling

Exhibit 18-2. Action Levels for Surface Sampling

Exhibit 20-1. Example Action Plan for Compliance with USP <797>

LIST OF TABLES

Tables are numbered consecutively throughout <797>.

Table 1. Action Level for Gloved Fingertip and Thumb Sampling

Table 2. ISO Classification of Particulate Matter in Room Air

Table 3. Summary of Minimum Requirements for Placement of PEC for Compounding Non-HD CSPs

Table 4. Summary of ACPH Requirements for Non-HD Sterile Compounding Areas

Table 5. Action Levels for Viable Airborne Particle Air Sampling

Table 6. Action Levels for Surface Sampling

Table 7. Purpose of Cleaning, Disinfecting, and Sporicidal Agents

Table 8. Minimum Frequency for Cleaning and Disinfecting Surfaces and Applying Sporicidal Agents in Classified Areas and Within the Perimeter of the SCA

Table 9. Summary of Terms

Table 10. BUDs for Category 1 CSPs

Table 11. BUDs for Category 2 CSPs

LIST OF BOXES

Boxes are numbered to match the section number; not every section has a box and some sections have multiple boxes.

Box 2-1. Gloved Fingertip and Thumb Sampling Procedures

Box 2-2. Media Fill Testing Procedures

Box 3-1. Hand Washing Procedures

Box 3-2. Hand Sanitizing Procedures

Box 6-1. Active Air Sampling Procedures for Viable Airborne Monitoring

Box 6-2. Surface Sampling Procedures

Box 7-1. Procedures for Cleaning and Disinfecting the PEC

Box 7-2. Procedures for Applying a Sporicidal Agent in the PEC

Box 11-1. Master Formulation Records

Box 11-2. Compounding Records

Box 21-1. Compounding Records for Individual Allergenic Extract Prescription Sets

USP <797> AVAILABILITY

1.1 Where can I find the full text of <797>?

United States Pharmacopeial Convention (USP) publishes the *USP Compounding Compendium*.[1] It contains all the major compounding chapters: *USP General Chapter <795> Pharmaceutical Compounding—Nonsterile Preparations*,[2] *USP General Chapter <797> Pharmaceutical Compounding—Sterile Preparation*,[3] *USP General Chapter <800> Hazardous Drugs—Handling in Healthcare Settings*,[4] and *USP General Chapter <825> Radiopharmaceuticals—Preparation, Compounding, Dispensing, and Repackaging*[5] as well as all the other chapters that are referenced in those core compounding chapters. Additionally, the General Notices that apply to compounding and compounding monographs are included. The *USP Compounding Compendium* is available through USP at www.usp.org as an annual subscription.

Your subscription allows you to download updates throughout your subscription year. Be sure to do that each February, June, and November so you have the most current versions of existing chapters and any new General Notices, General Chapters, or monographs that were completed in the prior months.

1.2 When did <797> become official?

<797> has been an official standard since 2004. It was revised in 2008. The most recent revision was published in June 2019 and becomes official when announced by USP.

1.3 Why is there a need for a chapter on sterile compounding? Is this all about the meningitis scare from 2012?

This is a focus on patient safety. It was first published in 2004, so <797> predates the meningitis tragedy of 2012. There were several issues of improper quality (strength as well as microbial contamination) that occurred in 1989 and 1990, prompting both a Food and Drug Administration (FDA) Alert and an ASHP Urgent Attention letter directed to sterile compounders.[6] Those events and others led to the development of <797>.

1.4 Is <797> a guideline? A requirement?

<797> is a minimum standard. Regulators such as federal or state entities can make it a regulation by including it in their documents. Accreditation organizations, such as The Joint Commission, DNV-GL Healthcare, the Pharmacy Compounding Accreditation Boards, and others, can include it in their own standards.

1.5 How can <797> be a minimum standard if my state hasn't incorporated it into regulations?

USP is a standard-setting organization. Even if your state has not codified it into regulation, it is still a federal standard and can be used to inspect or survey your pharmacy.

GENERAL PRINCIPLES OF USP <797>

2.1 Is this a new USP chapter?

The 2019 standard is a revision. <797> was first published in 2004. It was previously revised in 2008.

2.2 What are the major differences between the version of <797> that has been official for a while and the 2019 version of <797>?

You will notice that the arrangement of text of <797> is similar to that of *USP General Chapter <795> Pharmaceutical Compounding—Nonsterile Preparations.*[2] Details have been added incorporating evolving best practices. Updates include the following:

- Elimination of the risk levels (low, medium, high) of compounded sterile preparations (CSPs)
- Assignment of at least one designated person to oversee compounding activities
- Assignment of beyond-use dates (BUDs) based on the facility in which the CSP is mixed
- Changes in the BUDs (including a maximum number of days)
- Defined frequency of surface sampling (monthly)
- More details for procedures, such as media fill tests, gloved fingertip and thumb tests, and environmental monitoring

2.3 When must I comply with <797>?

<797> is an existing USP General Chapter, so compliance has been required since 2004. The latest revision was published on June 1, 2019. Federal and state regulators and accreditation organizations may incorporate USP standards in their own regulations and standards. Check with the organizations with jurisdiction over your site to be sure you comply with their requirements.

2.4 What is the distinction between the terms *must* and *should* in the text of <797>?

Yes. USP uses *must* for a requirement and *should* for a recommendation. However, some states may expect you to comply with recommendations as well as USP requirements. Consult your state regulations, which may be more stringent than the USP standard.

2.5 If I'm just repackaging sterile products into unit doses, do I need to comply with <797>?

Yes. Repackaging of sterile components is within the scope of <797>. See the FDA document on repackaging.[7]

2.6 Are hazardous drugs addressed in <797>?

Compounding sterile hazardous drugs must comply with both <797> and *USP General Chapter <800> Hazardous Drugs—Handling in Healthcare Settings*.[4] Also see *The Chapter <800> Answer Book*[8] for information on compounding sterile hazardous drugs.

2.7 Are radiopharmaceuticals addressed in <797>?

No. They are addressed in *USP General Chapter <825> Radiopharmaceuticals—Preparation, Compounding, Dispensing, and Repackaging*.[5]

2.8 Are allergens addressed in <797>?

Yes. Compounding allergenic extracts are within the scope of <797> and addressed in a section of the standard.

CONTENTS OF SECTIONS OF USP <797>

USP General Chapter <797> Pharmaceutical Compounding—Sterile Preparations is divided into sections. The key elements in each section are listed below.

Introduction and Scope
- Functions that are in and out of scope of <797>

Personnel Training and Evaluation
- Assignment of a person who is responsible for oversight of compounding in your organization
- Responsibilities of all personnel who compound sterile preparations
- Competency documentation required

Personal Hygiene and Garbing
- Activities prior to compounding
- Hand hygiene
- Required and recommended garb

Facilities and Engineering Controls
- Facility design requirements for compounding sterile drugs
- Secondary engineering controls
- Compounding suite
- Segregated compounding areas
- Primary engineering controls for compounding sterile drugs
  - Laminar air flow systems
  - Restricted access barrier systems
  - Pharmaceutical isolators

Certification and Recertification
- Monitoring particles and air flow

Microbiological Air and Surface Monitoring
- Appropriate media and devices for monitoring
- Electronic air monitoring
- Surface sampling

Cleaning, Disinfecting, and Applying Sporicidal Agents in Compounding Areas
- Selection of agents
- Steps in the cleaning process
- Minimum frequency of cleaning

Introducing Items into the Secondary and Primary Engineering Controls
- Movement of materials into the rooms and hoods

Equipment, Supplies, and Components
- Equipment used for compounding
- Ingredients used for compounding

Sterilization and Depyrogenation
- Terminal sterilization
- Filtration

Master Formulation and Compounding Records
- Creating and maintaining required records

Release Inspections and Testing
- Final checks of compounded sterile preparations (CSPs)
- Frequency of required sterility testing and endotoxins levels

Labeling
- Requirements for the label
- Requirement for additional labeling

Establishing Beyond-Use Dates
- How to calculate beyond-use dates

Use of Conventionally Manufactured Products as Components
- Using single-dose vials
- Using multiple-dose vials
- Using pharmacy bulk packages

Use of CSPs as Components
- Use of compounded preparations as an ingredient in another CSP

Standard Operating Procedures (SOPs)
- Establishing and following policies and procedures

Quality Assurance and Quality Control
- Process to ensure quality
- Evaluation of conditions that do not meet accepted standards

- Process to ensure addressing patient concerns

CSP Handling, Storage, Packaging, Shipping, and Transport
- Selection of packaging materials

Documentation
- Required documentation

Compounding Allergenic Extracts
- Facility design
- Personnel requirements

Glossary
- Definition of terms used in <797>

Appendix
- Acronyms used in <797>

LIST OF TABLES

Tables are numbered consecutively throughout <797>.

Table Number	Title
1	Action Level for Gloved Fingertip and Thumb Sampling
2	ISO Classification of Particulate Matter in Room Air
3	Summary of Minimum Requirements for Placement of PEC for Compounding Non-HD CSPs
4	Summary of ACPH Requirements for Non-HD Sterile Compounding Areas
5	Action Levels for Viable Airborne Particle Air Sampling
6	Action Levels for Surface Sampling
7	Purpose of Cleaning, Disinfecting, and Sporicidal Agents
8	Minimum Frequency for Cleaning and Disinfecting Surfaces and Applying Sporicidal Agents in Classified Areas and Within the Perimeter of the SCA
9	Summary of Terms
10	BUDs for Category 1 CSPs
11	BUDs for Category 2 CSPs

ACPH = air changes per hour, BUD = beyond-use date, CSP = compounded sterile preparation, HD = hazardous drug, PEC = primary engineering control, SCA = segregated compounding area.

LIST OF BOXES

Boxes are numbered to match the section number; not every section has a box and some sections have multiple boxes.

Box Number	Title
2-1	Gloved Fingertip and Thumb Sampling Procedures
2-2	Media Fill Testing Procedures
3-1	Hand Washing Procedures
3-2	Hand Sanitizing Procedures
6-1	Active Air Sampling Procedures for Viable Airborne Monitoring
6-2	Surface Sampling Procedures
7-1	Procedures for Cleaning and Disinfecting the PEC
7-2	Procedures for Applying a Sporicidal Agent in the PEC
11-1	Master Formulation Records
11-2	Compounding Records
21-1	Compounding Records for Individual Allergenic Extract Prescription Sets

PEC = primary engineering control.

SCOPE OF USP <797>

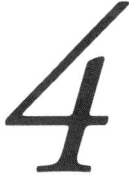

(See Section 1 in USP <797>.)

4.1 Who has to comply with <797>?

All healthcare personnel who compound sterile preparations.

4.2 I've heard <797> referred to as a guideline and a standard. Which is correct? What's the difference?

<797> is a federal standard. It's not a guideline; you cannot select certain aspects to consider. You need to follow the entire standard to be compliant.

4.3 Is <797> a regulation?

It is a federal standard. States and other regulatory agencies, accreditation organizations, and health-system policies may include <797> requirements.

4.4 Does <797> apply to animals?

Yes. It applies to sterile compounding for humans and animals.

4.5 Can I select certain sections of <797> to be compliant with?

No. You need to comply with the entire standard.

4.6 Is <797> in effect now?

Yes. It has been since 2004 and was revised in 2008. The most recent version was published on June 1, 2019 and becomes official when announced by USP.

4.7 What are examples of preparations that must comply—and those that do not comply—with <797>?

Sterile preparations include infusions, injections, inhalations, irrigations for internal body categories, ophthalmics (including drops), implants, and soaks for live organs and tissues. Prepackaging of sterile products and preparations also must comply with <797>. Compounding nasal dosage forms for local application or irrigations for the mouth, rectal cavity, or sinus cavity are not required to be sterile so must comply with <795>.[2]

4.8 Does <797> apply to all compounds?

It applies to all sterile compounds. Nonsterile compounds must comply with <795>.[2] Compounding with hazardous drugs —either nonsterile or sterile—must also comply with <800>.[4]

4.9 Does <797> apply to investigational agents?

Yes. if the investigational agent is a sterile compounded preparation. There is also a USP chapter that deals specifically with phase 1 studies: *USP General Chapter <1168> Compounding for Phase 1 Investigational Studies.*[9]

4.10 I work in a hospital pharmacy. Do I need to comply with <795> or <797>?

It depends on the type of preparation. For nonsterile preparations, use <795>. For sterile preparations, use <797>. For hazardous drug (HD) compounding, you also need to comply with <800>.

4.11 Does <800> replace <797>?

No. <800> provides the information on handling HDs. It must be used in conjunction with <797> for sterile compounding.

4.12 Do community or mail-order pharmacies have to comply with <797>? How about a private physician's office?

All healthcare sites where sterile compounding occurs must comply with <797>. This includes pharmacies of any type, physician offices and clinics, veterinarian offices, and any other healthcare setting where sterile preparations are compounded.

4.13 Do pharmaceutical manufacturers have to comply with <797>?

The scope of <797> is compounding. Manufacturers are under different—and more stringent—requirements to manufacture pharmaceutical products.

4.14 Does a nursing home have to comply with <797>?

The pharmacy provider should be preparing the compounded sterile preparations (CSPs) for the long-term care (LTC) facility. Generally, the activities at an LTC site are preparation per approved labeling, which is out of scope of <797> as long as the preparation is for a single patient and will not be stored. However, if sterile compounding is occurring at an LTC facility, those healthcare professionals need to comply with <797>.

4.15 What types of activities aren't considered compounding?

If you dispense a conventionally manufactured product without having to manipulate it prior to dispensing, it's not compounding. Preparing doses using manufacturer's instructions for administration to a single patient right away isn't compounding.

4.16 How is administering medications distinguished from compounding?

If a dose is prepared for administration (such as by using the manufacturer's instructions) and administered within 4 hours of preparation, it does not meet the definition of compounding. An example of "Immediate Use" might be an ICU nurse preparing a sodium bicarbonate drip for a stat dose. Although neither need to meet the requirements for Category 1 or 2 CSPs (see Section 11), they still need to be mixed using aseptic technique.

4.17 I thought medications had to be administered within 1 hour of compounding. Which is correct: within 1 hour or within 4 hours?

The 2008 version of <797> used 1 hour as the time limit between immediate-use preparation of a CSP and the start of administration of the CSP. That time has been changed to 4 hours in the 2019 version of <797>. 2019 revisions of <795> and <797> both include the 4-hour limit. However, most health systems are likely to continue using a 1-hour limit because this meets the needs of patient care while maintaining the patient safety aspects of pharmacy preparation of compounds (both nonsterile and sterile). Areas such as surgical services may the need 4-hour allowance.

4.18 Does <797> include prepackaging from a vial to a unit-dose syringe?

Yes. That meets the definition of compounding in <797>.

4.19 <795> says repackaging is out of scope. Why is it included in <797>?

<797> deals with stability (drug, diluent, container, closure) as well as sterility. Repackaging of a sterile product or preparation from one container to another needs to include the assessment of the change of the container (e.g., vial to syringe) and closure (e.g., manufacturer's vial closure to syringe cap).

4.20 Is it OK to compound a preparation that can be mixed cheaper than the commercial product?

No, if only for the cost issue. See the FDA guidance document *Compounded Drug Products That Are Essentially Copies of Commercially Available Drug Products* under Section 503A of the Federal Food, Drug, and Cosmetic Act.[10]

4.21 Who will enforce <797> for compliance outside of pharmacy settings?

A federal agency can. States determine how they will enforce any standards. Most states have had regulations related to nonsterile compounding for decades and have recently added regulations related to sterile compounding. Accreditation organizations have incorporated <797> in their standards.

HUMAN RESOURCES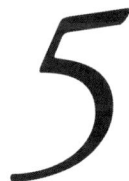

(See Section 2 in USP <797>.)

5.1 DESIGNATED PERSON

5.1-1 Who is the designated person mentioned in <797>?

Each compounding site must have one or more individuals assigned who oversees the responsibilities of compounding sterile preparations. These individuals are responsible for developing and implementing policies and procedures; overseeing compliance with <797> and any other applicable laws, regulations, and standards; ensuring competency of personnel; and ensuring environmental control of the facilities used for storing and compounding CSPs.

5.1-2 Can the designated person be a committee instead of an individual?

There needs to be at least one person identified. That person can lead a committee if that approach is chosen by the entity or could oversee other designated persons.

5.1-3 Does the designated person need to be a pharmacist?

No. It can be anyone qualified to perform the required functions. Healthcare systems will most likely have a pharmacist in this position, but some organizations may assign a pharmacy technician to that function if permitted by state regulations. Some entities (e.g., physician offices, veterinary clinics) may not have a pharmacist available for this function, so will need to assign a qualified person to oversee the compounding functions.

5.1-4 Does the designated person need to be a manager?

No. It is up to the entity to assign the specific person to oversee this.

5.1-5 Is the designated person responsible for compliance with <797>?

Yes. It is a key function of the designated person.

5.1-6 Does oversight of sterile compounding have to be the designated person's sole job responsibility?

No. It is up to the organization to assign job functions.

5.1-7 Can the designated person be responsible for more than one site?

Yes. It is up to the entity to assign the responsibility. One person can have responsibility for multiple sites. In multihospital health systems, it is likely that one person would be responsible for oversight of multiple hospitals and other sites that compound.

5.1-8 Where can the designated person obtain the necessary training for this job?

That is up to the entity to define. Training needs to include both didactic and hands-on experience. ASHP offers a certificate program on sterile compounding.[11] CriticalPoint[12] offers didactic and hands-on training.

5.1-9 How much training does the designated person need to have?

<797> does not specify the number of hours. Some state regulations require a specific number for relicensure of pharmacists and/or other compounders. The designated person must have a thorough understanding of the standards to be able to develop, implement, and oversee policies, procedures, and practices including personnel training, evaluation, and monitoring as well as facility compliance with <797> and other laws and regulations.

5.1-10 What types of activities is the designated person typically responsible for?

Items include the following:

- Compliance with <797>, applicable federal and state laws and regulations, and accreditation standards
- Oversight of personnel training, competency documentation, and monitoring
- Oversight of facility use and monitoring
- Establish standard operating procedures (SOPs)
- Develop master formulation records
- Monitor beyond-use dates

5.1-11 Does the designated person need to be board-certified?

It is up to the entity to define the requirements. The Board of Pharmacy Specialties (BPS) Compounded Sterile Preparations Pharmacist (BCSCP) is a criterion that could be applied.[13] If the designated person is a pharmacy technician, the Pharmacy Technician Certification Board (PTCB) additional distinction of Certified Compounded Sterile Preparation Technician™ (CSPT™) is available and could be included as a criterion.[14] Other certificate programs such as ASHP's Sterile Products Preparation Certificate Program,[11] CriticalPoint LLC's Qualified Person Certification[12] could also be used as a criterion.

5.2 RESPONSIBILITIES OF COMPOUNDING PERSONNEL

5.2-1 What training is required for compounding CSPs?

Education and training concerning sterile compounding need to supplement general education, training, and documentation of competency for handling any drug. *Competence Assessment Tools for Health-System Pharmacies*[15] and ASHP's *Pharmacy Competency Assessment Center*[16] provides checklists and competence documents, including one for compounding sterile preparations. All personnel compounding CSPs need to complete training such as organizational policies and procedures, use of garb, use of equipment, selection of components, and spill management. Personnel must document competency prior to independently compounding CSPs for patients. Competency in hand hygiene and successful completion of media fill and gloved fingertip and thumb testing must be done every 6 months. Other competency must be documented at least every 12 months.

5.2-2 What are the key competencies that compounders must demonstrate?

<797> lists the core competencies required, including hand hygiene, garbing, knowledge of compounding technique, proper movement of materials, cleaning and disinfection, calculations, measuring and mixing, aseptic technique, achieving and maintaining sterility and apyrogenicity, proper use of equipment, and documentation[3].

5.3 DOCUMENTING COMPETENCE

5.3-1 What competence information has to be documented?

Competence documents must show that the person can perform functions of the position and that they will comply with your organizational policies and procedures. *Competence Assessment Tools for Health-System Pharmacies*[15] and ASHP's *Pharmacy Competency Assessment Center*[16] provides compounding-related assessments and forms. Compounding requires observation by skilled personnel to ensure proper techniques are followed; be sure to document this observational review and approval. Regulatory inspectors and accreditation organization surveyors often expect tests to have a designated passing score defined in policy.

5.3-2 How often should training occur?

Initial training needs to be completed prior to independently compounding CSPs for patients. Ongoing education and training need to occur whenever new procedures or new equipment is used. Visual observation of hand hygiene and garbing, successful completion of the requalifying gloved fingertip and thumb test, and successful completion of a media fill test must occur every 6 months. Documentation of ongoing competence for other core competencies needs to occur at least every 12 months.

5.3-3 Is there a set number of training hours required?

There is no such requirement in <797> although some states have a minimum number of training hours in their regulations.

5.3-4 Do pharmacists who only check—but don't compound—CSPs have to document competency?

Yes. There is no "just checking" with compounding. Whoever is checking needs to be fully competent to perform compounding, so they know what they are checking. They need to complete all the required tests at the same frequency as any personnel who compound CSPs.

5.3-5 I am at a small hospital and the only pharmacist. How can I document my competency?

You could attend an external training program or have a competent trainer provide education at your site.

5.4 HAZARD COMMUNICATION PLAN

> All entities must have a hazard communication plan. This is a requirement of the Occupational Safety and Health Administration (OSHA).

5.4-1 What is a hazard communication plan?

OSHA requires all workplaces where employees are exposed to hazardous chemicals to have a written plan describing how the standard will be implemented in that facility.[17]

5.4.2 Is a hazardous chemical the same thing as a hazardous drug?

Not necessarily. The hazardous drugs (HDs) defined in <800> are those in the National Institute for Occupational Safety and Health (NIOSH) list of HDs.[18] OSHA's hazardous chemical standard includes much more than the NIOSH list because it deals with all types of hazardous chemicals, not just those that are hazardous to healthcare personnel. Review the safety data sheets (SDSs) for chemicals used for compounding and cleaning.

5.4-3 Where can I find safety data sheets?

OSHA requires that chemical manufacturers, distributors, or importers of the hazardous material provide detailed information on the product. SDSs—formerly called material safety data sheets (MSDSs)—provide a structured document that includes the required information you need. You may need to request an SDS from the supplier.

5.4-4 Do all drugs require an SDS?

The raw chemical may, but some dosage forms are exempt from the requirement.

SDSs are required for the following:

- Drugs deemed hazardous by the manufacturer
- Solid medications that contain hazardous substances that are intended to be dissolved or crushed before administration

SDSs are not required for the following:

- Medications that don't contain hazardous substances
- Medications that are in solid, final form for direct administration to the patient
- Drugs packaged by the manufacturer for sale to consumers (like over-the-counter medications)

See the OSHA Hazard Communication Standard for further information.[17]

5.4-5 Whose responsibility is it to develop a hazard communication plan?

In a health system, this likely is a function of the Safety Department or other similar department. For small employers that need a summary document, see OSHA's Hazard Communication: *Small Entity Compliance Guide for Employers That Use Hazardous Chemicals*.[19]

POLICIES AND PROCEDURES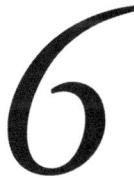

(See Sections 17 and 20 in USP <797>.)

6.1 What type of policies should I have?

See **Exhibit 6-1.** Your state, accreditation organization, or other agency may require additional policies.

6.2 Are SOPs and policies the same thing?

Yes. SOP is an acronym for standard operating procedures.

6.3 Do the policies have to be written?

Yes. The format is up to you; they can be hard copy or electronic. The key requirement is that they are retrievable.

6.4 Who, and at what frequency, needs to review policies?

Policies need to be reviewed as new compounds are made, new equipment is used, or other situations that warrant a review. Minimally, the designated person needs to review policies every 12 months.

6.5 How long do I have to keep old policies?

At least 3 years or longer if required by your jurisdiction, inspecting agency, accreditation organization, or health-system policy.

EXHIBIT 6-1. Policies Required and Recommended in USP <797>

Note: If hazardous drugs are compounded, additional policies and procedures are required. See <800>[4] and *The Chapter <800> Answer Book*.[8]

- Designated person(s)
  - Qualification and training
  - Identification of specific individuals
  - Responsibilities
- Develop and implement policies and procedures
- Oversee organizational compliance with <797> and other applicable laws, regulations, and standards
- Ensure competency of personnel
- Ensure environmental control of the storage and compounding areas
- Understand rationale for risk-prevention policies and risks to personnel
- Report potentially unsafe or hazardous situations to the management team
- Monitor the compounding area
  - Daily activities
  - Semiannual certification
  - Environmental monitoring plan
  - Corrective action plan for excursions
- Monitor and observe compounding activities and personnel
- Maintain reports of testing and sampling performed and act on the results
- Hazard communication program related to compounding
- Personnel training
  - Compliance with appropriate USP standards for compounding standards
  - Proper use of garb and frequency of changing components
  - Proper use of equipment and components
  - Use of aseptic and other appropriate technique
  - Spill management
  - Proper disposal
- Hand hygiene
- Proper use of garb
  - Gloves, gowns, masks, hair/head covers, shoe covers
  - Other required garb components
  - Frequency of changing garb
  - Disposal of used garb

EXHIBIT 6-1. (cont'd)

- Personnel responsibilities
  - Understand the fundamental practices and precautions
  - Continually evaluate procedures and the quality of compounded sterile preparations (CSPs) to prevent harm to patients
- Designation of compounding areas
  - Restricted access to only authorized personnel
  - Sterile compounding area
  - Sterile compounding suite (anteroom + buffer room)
  - Segregated compounded area
  - Acceptable temperature and humidity ranges and pressure gradients and action to take it out of range
- Receiving and unpacking components
- Storage
  - Not stored on the floor
  - Meets applicable safety precautions
  - Meets temperature requirements (i.e., room, refrigerator, freezer, warmer) and addresses temperature excursions
- Compounding area
  - Surfaces of ceilings, walls, floors, fixtures, shelving, counters, and cabinets must be smooth, impervious, free from cracks and crevices, nonshedding, and able to withstand decontamination and cleaning
  - Sink and eyewash location—no closer than 1 meter to any primary engineering control or entrance to any negative pressure area, and the buffer room cannot contain any water sources
  - If nonsterile compounding is done in a biological safety cabinet (BSC) used for sterile compounding, nonsterile compounding cannot occur when sterile compounding is occurring
- Equipment records
  - Primary engineering controls and other classified areas must be certified every 6 months using the elements listed in the Controlled Environment Testing Association (CETA) guidance documents
- Components
  - Receipt of components
  - Certificates of analysis
  - Safety data sheets for active pharmaceutical ingredients and how to retrieve and interpret them
- Compounding
  - Master formulation records
  - Compounding records
  - Release inspection and testing

EXHIBIT 6-1. (cont'd)

- Beyond-use dates
- Labeling CSPs
- Packaging CSPs
  - Safe work practices
- Cleaning and sanitizing
  - Cleaning—solutions used and procedure
  - Application of sterile isopropyl alcohol to surfaces
- Waste segregation and disposal
  - Applicable federal, state, and local information and organizational policy
- Quality assurance/quality control
  - Roles, duties, and training for each aspect of the quality assurance/quality control (QA/QC) program
  - Complaint receipt, acknowledgment, and handling
  - Results of investigation and corrective action

GARB AND HAND HYGIENE

(See Section 3 in USP <797>.)

7.1 GENERAL INFORMATION

7.1-1   What does <797> require for garb?

The components of required garb include gowns, gloves, hair covers, masks, and shoe covers. If you are compounding hazardous compounded sterile preparationss (CSPs), additional personal protective equipment (PPE) is required. See <800>[4] and *The Chapter <800> Answer Book*[8] for details.

The garbing procedure—the order in which garb is donned—needs to be developed and detailed in your policies and needs to match the facility design (such as placement of the sink) you have.

7.1-2   What is the purpose of garb?

Garb provides protection for the preparation you are compounding.

7.1-3   What is the difference between garb and PPE?

Think of *garb* as protection for the preparation you are compounding and *PPE* as protection for the compounder.

7.1-4   Is different garb required for hazardous and nonhazardous CSPs?

Some of the components are the same, such as hair covers, shoe covers, and masks. Specific types of gloves and gowns must be worn when mixing antineoplastics (and other hazardous drugs if they are not entity-exempt through the organization's Assessment of Risk). See <800>[4] and *The Chapter <800> Answer Book*[8] for details for PPE requirements and recommendations when compounding hazardous drugs. Chemotherapy (commonly known as "chemo") gowns and sterile chemo gloves can be used when compounding nonhazardous CSPs, but they also need to meet the requirements of garb for compounding nonhazardous CSPs.

7.1-5   Is additional garb required for personnel who are compounding from powders?

This needs to be addressed in your policies and procedures. There is additional eye and respiratory risk when working with active pharmaceutical ingredients (APIs) and other raw materials.

7.1-6 Do I need to wear garb if the hood I work in is a glove box?

Yes. Compounding isolators require the same garb as used when working in traditional laminar air flow workbenches.

7.1-7 What does *donning* and *doffing* mean?

Don means to put on PPE; *doff* means to remove it.

7.1-8 Does the pharmacist who is only checking items need to garb?

It depends on the location where checking occurs. Whoever is in the sterile compounding area needs to be appropriately garbed. It doesn't matter if they are compounding, checking, observing, certifying, cleaning, repairing equipment, or any other activity.

7.1-9 Can garb be reused?

Gowns used for nonhazardous compounding—if not soiled or contaminated—can be carefully removed and hung up inside the anteroom or segregated compounding area (SCA) for use for the remainder of the shift. Other disposable garb must not be reused. Reusable garb (such as goggles) must be cleaned and disinfected after use.

7.1-10 The pharmacists and technicians who work in our operating room (OR) satellite wear "OR greens." Is this sufficient garb?

It depends what they are doing. If you are preparing intravenous (IV) mixtures in an SCA, you need the additional garb required. If you are mixing an IV for immediate use, it may be sufficient based on your policies

7.2 HAND HYGIENE

7.2-1 What does *hand hygiene* mean?

The Centers for Disease Control and Prevention (CDC) defines *hand hygiene* as "cleaning your hands by using either handwashing (washing hands with soap and water), antiseptic hand wash, antiseptic hand rub (i.e., alcohol-based hand sanitizer including foam or gel), or surgical hand antisepsis." Prior to compounding, you need to wash your hands with soap and water. Use of only alcohol hand sanitizers is not enough. See the CDC's Hand Hygiene in Healthcare Settings[20] guidelines for further information.

7.2-2 Can alcohol-based hand gel be used instead of soap and water?

No. It is not a replacement for soap and water. Alcohol-based hand gel is used as part of the hand hygiene and garbing procedure.

7.2-3 How long should our policy say to wash hands?

Prior to compounding, wash your hands and forearms with soap and water for at least 30 seconds.

7.2-4 Are regular paper towels OK to use?

No. Use low-linting disposable towels or wipers.

7.3 GLOVES

7.3-1 When gloves are mentioned in <797>, what kind of gloves does that mean?

Sterile, powder-free gloves. If hazardous CSPs are compounded, gloves that meet ASTM Standard D6978 are required.

7.3-2 Is it OK to wash gloves between compounds?

No. If gloves are soiled or contaminated, they need to be discarded and new gloves donned.

7.3-3 When are sterile gloves required?

Sterile gloves are required when compounding CSPs.

7.3-4 We use glove boxes to put on gloves outside of the glove box. Is this correct?

No. When using compounding isolators, you need to pass the sterile gloves through the antechamber and don them inside the compounding aseptic isolator (CAI) or compounding aseptic containment isolator (CACI) over the gloves on the compounding isolator sleeves.

7.3-5 Are sterile gloves required when working in a compounding isolator?

Yes. A sterile glove needs to be the one that touches the preparation. *You need a minimum of two pairs of gloves:* one on the compounding isolator sleeve (that is changed at least daily) and another pair for the compounder. Those gloves must be passed through the antechamber and donned inside the CAI. You may also want to use another disposable pair of gloves to use on your hands inside the gloves accessed through the compounding isolator sleeve.

7.3-6 How often do compounding isolator gloves need to be changed?

The gloves connected to the sleeves need to be changed at least daily or if they are torn or punctured or if you know or suspect they have been contaminated. They also need to be changed if compounders use different size gloves so their gloves would not fit over the CAI gloves.

7.3-7 Do chemo gloves have to meet a particular standard?

Yes. Chemotherapy ("chemo") gloves used for handling hazardous drugs (HDs) must meet ASTM Standard D6978, the *Standard Practice for Assessment of Resistance of Medical Gloves to Permeation by Chemotherapy Drugs.*[21] Some gloves are tested only for permeation to general chemicals using ASTM Standard F739-99a (*Standard Test Method for Resistance of Protective Clothing Materials to Permeation by Liquids or Gases under Conditions of Continuous Contact*[22]), which is not sufficient for HD gloves.

7.3-8 How do I know if a glove is chemo-rated?

Documentation that the gloves meet ASTM D6978 needs to be listed on the product labeling. It can generally be found on the box of the gloves.

7.3-9 Is it OK for chemo gloves to be tested per ASTM D6978 and laboratory chemical tested per ASTM F739?

Yes, as long as they document that they meet the ASTM Standard D6978.

7.4 GOWNS

7.4-1 Do gowns have to be sterile?

<797> does not require sterile gowns.

7.4-2 What is the difference between gowns we use for non-HDs and those used for chemo?

Gowns used for handling antineoplastic agents must be impervious. Gowns used for non-HDs can be made of other materials, depending on their intended use. Your entity's Assessment of Risk may allow different gowns when handling HDs that are not National Institute for Occupational Safety and Health (NIOSH) Table 1 antineoplastic agents.[18]

7.4-3 Can I hang my gown in the anteroom for use later in the day?

Yes, if it was used for nonhazardous drug preparation and is not soiled or otherwise compromised. If your policy allows, you can reuse the gown within the same shift as long as it is hung inside the classified area or inside the perimeter of the SCA. Gowns used to mix chemo cannot be reused.

7.4-4 Are washable gowns OK to use?

Yes, if they are low-linting, have sleeves that fit snugly around the wrist, and are enclosed at the neck. However, consider use of disposable gowns. If you use washable gowns, a clean gown needs to be donned daily and whenever soiled or contaminated.

7.4-5 Do I need to wear a regular gown under my chemo gown?

That is not specified in <797>, but think about your facility design and work practices. If you are in a sterile compounding suite, you need to have a regular gown under your chemo gown because you will be entering the clean side of your anteroom when you exit your negative pressure buffer room. You have to be properly gowned at that point, so you need to have on a gown, gloves, mask, hair cover, and shoe covers.

If your HD facility is a containment segregated compounding area (C-SCA) or an area devoted to nonsterile compounding, you may not need a regular gown because you will be exiting into a general pharmacy area. However, think of your containment practices. Consider using a regular gown even in these situations to further protect your clothing.

7.5 HAIR COVERS

7.5-1 What is the difference between head and beard covers used for chemo and those used for nonhazardous CSPs?

There is no difference. The same products can be used for handling HDs as you use for handling non-HDs.

7.5-2 One of our employees is completely bald. Does he need to wear a hair cover?

Yes. It's to cover the head as well as hair. Humans still shed particles, and that's what head and hair covers are intended to mitigate.

7.5-3 If personnel wear a head cover for religious or other reasons, is an additional hair cover necessary?

Yes. The purpose of the hair covers is to protect the preparation from potential microbial contamination. Hair covers come in various formats, including bouffants and hoods. The additional head/hair covers must be placed over the head cover worn for religious or other reasons.

7.5-4 Do earrings have to be removed, or can they just be covered by the hair cover?

They need to be removed. <797> requires removal of piercings that could interfere with the effectiveness of garbing. Earrings could get caught on the hair cover, and they also could be a contamination risk.

7.6 MASKS

7.6-1 Do I have to wear a surgical mask when compounding?

A surgical or procedural mask is required for sterile compounding. However, a mask is *not* respiratory protection; it protects the preparation, not the compounder.

7.6-2 Is a mask the same thing as a respirator?

No. The surgical or procedural mask is worn to protect the preparation you are mixing. It does not protect your respiratory system. A respirator, which also functions as a mask, provides respiratory protection to the compounder.

7.6-3 Is a face shield a mask?

They are not the same. You still need a mask when wearing a face shield, unless you use a combined mask/face shield.

7.7 SLEEVES

7.7-1 Are sleeve covers required?

No, but they can be used if required by your policy.

7.8 SHOE COVERS

7.8-1 What is the difference between shoe covers used for chemo and those used for non-HDs?

There is no difference. The same products can be used for handling HDs as you use for handling non-HDs. However, you may want to consider using shoe covers that are impervious.

7.8-2 Can I use dedicated cleanroom shoes instead of shoe covers?

No. You need to use shoe covers even if you have dedicated shoes for your cleanroom.

7.9 EYE PROTECTION

7.9-1 What does *eye protection* mean?

When eye protection is needed, it needs to be provided by using goggles. Goggles fit tightly, covering the eyes, eye sockets, and facial area surrounding the eyes. Goggles can be obtained that fit over eyeglasses.

7.9-2 I wear prescription eyeglasses. Does this qualify as eye protection?

No. Eyeglasses alone do not protect against splashes to the eyes. You need to obtain goggles that fit over your eyeglasses if eye protection is needed.

7.9-3 I wear a face shield to protect my contact lenses from drying out. Is this proper eye protection?

Face shields can be used to supplement other garb as long as it is not prohibited by your policy. Face shields alone do not protect against splashes to the eyes. You have to wear goggles when eye protection is needed.

7.9-4 Do I need eye protection when I'm cleaning up a spill?

Yes. Wear eye protection when cleaning up a spill.

7.10 RESPIRATORY PROTECTION

7.10-1 What does *respiratory protection* mean?

When respiratory protection is needed, a fit-tested NIOSH-certified N95 or more protective respirator is generally adequate to protect against airborne particles. However, N95 respirators don't protect against gases or vapors and provide only limited protection against direct liquid splashes. See the NIOSH page on Respiratory Trusted-Source Information[23] for more information.

7.10-2 What does an N95 respirator protect against?

It provides protection against airborne particles. It does not protect against gases or vapors.

7.10-3 Are there respirators that are better protection than N95?

There are other respirators that may meet your needs, which you should determine at your organization. Other types include full face-piece, chemical cartridge-type respirators, elastomeric half-mask respirators with multigas cartridges and P100 filters (or a cartridge targeted to the specific drug), or powered air purifying respirators (PAPRs).

7.10-4 Do surgical masks provide adequate respiratory protection?

Surgical or procedural masks do not provide respiratory protection from drug exposure and must not be used alone when respiratory protection is required.

7.10-5 Because the biological safety cabinet (BSC) and CACI provide respiratory protection, do I need to wear a regular mask for any HD compounding?

Yes. You need a surgical or procedural mask when compounding any sterile preparation.

7.10-6 Do I need respiratory protection when I'm cleaning up a spill?

Yes. Respiratory protection is needed when cleaning up a spill. Your policy needs to define the PPE required when cleaning up a spill.

7.11 GARBING PROCEDURES

7.11-1 What garb components are garbed first?

The order of garbing depends on the placement of your sink and your workflow. It needs to be defined to minimize potential contamination. Your policy needs to clearly list the components and order of garbing. Personnel need to be observed at least every 6 months to ensure they are correctly garbing and the review needs to be documented.

7.11-2 We put on hair covers, shoe covers, and masks before entering the clean side of the anteroom. In what order should these be donned?

It doesn't matter (unless required by your state), but the order must be detailed in your policy and followed. The order of garbing depends on the location of your sink and your workflow. Many organizations enter the dirty side of the anteroom, don these three components of garb, then step over into the clean side of the anteroom to wash hands, don gown, use alcohol-based hand rub on hands, and then don sterile gloves. Define the components of garb and order of garbing in your policy, and be sure the policy is followed by all who enter the compounding area.

7.11-3 What is the proper order of donning garb for compounding CSPs in a cleanroom suite (positive pressure anteroom with sink on the clean side of the anteroom and positive pressure buffer room)?

Your policies and procedures need to describe the garbing sequence based on your facility design.

To don garb for the facility design described in the question:

1. Enter dirty side of anteroom.
2. Don mask, hair cover, and shoe covers.
3. Step over into clean side of anteroom.
4. Wash hands.
5. Don gown.
6. Apply alcohol-based hand rub.
7. Don sterile gloves.

7.11-4 What is the proper order of donning garb for compounding CSPs in an SCA with a sink inside the room but outside the perimeter around the PEC?

Your policies and procedures need to describe the garbing sequence based on your facility design.

To don garb for the facility design described in the question:

1. Enter SCA, remaining outside the perimeter around the PEC.
2. Don mask, hair cover, and shoe covers.
3. Wash hands.
4. Don gown.
5. Step over the perimeter line.
6. Apply alcohol-based hand rub.
7. Don sterile gloves.

7.11-5 My facility design is different from the two examples above. Do I need to use only the order listed?

No. Your garbing procedure needs to match the design of your facility, particularly the location of your sink. Don garb in an order that reduces the risk of contamination.

7.11-6 Is additional garb required for personnel who are compounding from powders?

This should be considered in your policies and practices. There is additional eye and respiratory risk when working with APIs and other raw materials.

8 IMMEDIATE USE AND PREPARATION FOR ADMINISTRATION

(See Section 1 in USP <797>.)

8.1 What is considered *immediate use*?

Compounding that will be done immediately prior to administering the CSP to a patient does not necessarily need to comply with the facility or monitoring requirements detailed in <797>. Of course, for patient safety and consistency, it should if possible, but <797> allows for this for patient care needs. Acute care situations present where doses are needed stat for critical patients or a CSP is needed during a procedure that was unanticipated.

All of the following conditions must be met for a CSP to be considered immediate use:

- Written procedures are in place.
- The personnel mixing immediate-use preparations are aware of the organization's limited policies and have documented competence to comply with the policies.
- Aseptic procedures are followed.
- Compatibility of the components are known.
- Single-dose containers must be used for only one patient and cannot be saved for future use.
- The CSP is labeled, including the ingredients, preparer, and beyond-use time (which cannot exceed 4 hours from the time of preparation).

8.2 What is considered *administration*?

<797> is about compounding, so administration of medications is not in scope of the chapter. <797> defines *administration* as "the direct application of a sterile medication to a single patient by injecting, infusing, or otherwise providing a sterile medication in its final form."[3]

The information in the Centers for Disease Control and Prevention (CDC) Safe Injection Practices document[24] and related references should be used to establish the organization's policies concerning administration of sterile products and preparations.

8.3 What is considered *preparation for administration*?

Medications such as injections often contain instructions for preparation in FDA-approved labeling. This applies only to those medications that will be prepared for a single dose for a single patient that will be used right away and the specific instructions in the labeling are used. To meet this provision, the labeling must include the amount of the specific diluent to use, the strength of the final concentration, the type of container to use (such as a syringe or an IV bag), and the storage time allowed. If these details are not available, the full information in <797> must be followed.

8.4 Can nurses mix compounded sterile preparations (CSPs) for immediate use?

Yes. Any qualified health professional can mix an immediate-use preparation as long as it is within their scope of practice, your policy allows it, and they have documented competency.

8.5 Can staff other than nurses mix CSPs for immediate use?

Yes. Any qualified health professional can mix an immediate-use preparation as long as it is within their scope of practice, your policy allows it, and they have documented competency.

8.6 Can pharmacy personnel mix CSPs for immediate use?

Yes. Any qualified health professional can mix an immediate-use preparation as long as your policy allows, and they have documented competency.

8.7 Is reconstitution of an antibiotic vial considered immediate use or preparation for administration?

It depends on what is done with the reconstituted drug. If given immediately as an injection, it is preparation for administration. If mixed into an IV solution, using specific instructions in the product labeling include the specific diluent, IV solution base, and final concentration, it is *immediate use*. From a practical perspective in this situation, it depends on the limitations of your organizational policy.

8.8 Is there any difference between the previous definition of immediate use and the definition in the revised <797>?

There are two significant changes:

2008 version of <797>	2019 revision of <797>
Not more than three commercially manufactured sterile containers and not more than two entries into any one container	Not more than three different sterile products
Administration must begin within 1 hour	Administration must begin with 4 hours

8.9 What's the difference between using three sterile containers and using three different sterile products?

Here's an example: a nurse in the intensive care unit (ICU) needs to mix three vials of sodium bicarbonate into a liter bag of an IV solution for a stat dose. This would have violated the 2008 version of <797> because it would involve four containers (one IV bag + three vials of drug) and would have violated the number of entries into the IV bag (three from the three vials). This mixture is permitted under the 2019 revision of <797> because it involves two different products (the IV bag and the drug).

8.10 How long after someone mixes an immediate-use IV does it have to be used?

Administration of the CSP must be started within 4 hours of mixing. However, the 1-hour time has worked well for acute care hospitals, so there is no reason to change the policy because of the change allowed in the revision.

8.11 The previous version of <797> required that an immediate-use IV was hung within 1 hour of preparation. The revision says 4 hours. Which is correct?

The 2019 revision allows administration up to 4 hours after mixing. However, the 1-hour time has worked well for acute care hospitals in most cases. There is no requirement to change the policy because of the change allowed in the revision.

8.12 I thought immediate use meant to use it right away. Do we have to use a 4-hour beyond-use date for these IVs?

It does mean to use it right away. The immediate use provision is included in <797> to allow for the stat doses that are required for patient care. Because <797> applies to all sites where CSPs are made, there may be some procedural or nonacute sites where some additional time is necessary.

8.13 Can a Banana Bag be mixed under the immediate-use definition?

It depends on the content. Generally, such a mixture includes a base solution, folic acid, thiamine, and multiple vitamins. If that is the case, that is four components so outside of the definition of immediate use. Many organizations have approached this situation by running the thiamine via a secondary IV for the first bag then mixing subsequent bags under the requirements that meet either Category 1 or Category 2 CSPs. (See Section 11.)

8.14 Is it OK to let the night nursing supervisors enter the pharmacy to use the IV hood?

Why do you need to do that? Nursing can mix the IVs necessary for immediate use without the need to access the sterile compounding area. If they do use the hood, they need to comply with all the requirements of compounding personnel.

8.15 Our pharmacy is not open 24 hours. The nurses in ICU occasionally need to mix a sodium bicarbonate IV stat. Is this OK using the immediate-use definition?

Yes, as long as they have documented competency, organizational policy allows it, and the CSP contains no more than three different sterile products.

8.16 When anesthesia staff prepare syringes for cases, is this the immediate-use provision?

If syringes are prepared for a case outside of the facility conditions required for Category 1 or Category 2 medications (see Section 11), they need to meet the definition of preparation for administration, administration, or immediate use. As long as the drug is stable in the container and closure system used (e.g., syringe) and hospital policy permits, a 4-hour beyond-use time can be assigned.

8.17 Do nurses and anesthesia personnel need to complete the same competency to mix IVs that pharmacists and pharmacy techs need to do?

If they mix only immediate-use CSPs, they do not need to complete the media fill and gloved fingertip and thumb personnel requirements. However, they must have documented competence to mix immediate-use CSPs.

8.18 Do personnel who prepare only immediate-use IVs need to complete a media fill and gloved fingertip and thumb test?

If they mix only immediate-use CSPs, they do not need to complete the media fill and gloved fingertip and thumb personnel requirements. However, they must have documented competence to mix immediate-use CSPs.

8.19 Our pre-op area spikes a case of liters of Lactated Ringers for the following morning use. Is this OK under the immediate-use provision?

No. IV bags are single-use containers that do not contain preservatives. Administration is out of scope of <797> but consider the infection control risks. See the Association for Professionals in Infection Control and Epidemiology (APIC) position paper on Safe Infection, Infusion, and Medication Vial Practices in Healthcare[25] for further information.

8.20 One of our physicians is a dermatologist. Her staff prepares buffered lidocaine syringes for the day's use. Is this OK under the immediate-use provision?

It might be. See the definition of immediate use to be sure the preparation meets the definition. An entire day's worth would not be acceptable because there is a limit of 4 hours between mixing and administration.

8.21 One of our physician's offices has an allergy clinic. His staff mixes allergen extracts for patient use. Is this OK under the immediate-use provision?

The immediate-use provision doesn't apply in this situation, but there is a section in <797> that deals with requirements for preparation of allergen extracts. (See Section 11.4 and the information in Section 21 in <797>.)

PERSONNEL TRAINING AND COMPETENCE DOCUMENTATION

9

(See Sections 2 and 20 in USP <797>.)

9.1 INITIAL TRAINING

9.1-1 What initial training is required to mix compounded sterile preparations (CSPs)?

Personnel must be trained by a qualified person. A number of core competencies are required by <797>, and you will need to supplement those with your organizational-specific requirements.

9.1-2 What are the core competencies that a compounder must demonstrate?

Include these items in the training:
- Hand hygiene
- Garbing
- Calculations
- Measuring and mixing
- Moving products and supplies throughout the compounding space
- Aseptic technique
- Negative pressure technique (if hazardous drugs are compounded)
- Use of primary engineering controls
- Maintenance of secondary engineering controls
- Use of closed system drug-transfer devices (if used)
- Use of equipment and supplies
- Theoretical principles of air flow
- Use of autoclaves (if nonsterile-to-sterile preparations are mixed)
- Required documentation
- Cleaning and disinfection

9.1-3 Should I hire only personnel with prior IV room experience?

That is up to you, but you need to be sure that any personnel who compound are competent to do so. *Competency* is a combination of demonstration of core and other competencies, completion of the media fill and gloved fingertip and thumb tests, and knowledge of your organizational policies and procedures.

9.1-4 If people have documented training from other hospitals, do I need to train them?

Yes. They must be able to demonstrate successful completion of the same competencies you require for any compounder and demonstrate knowledge of your organizational policies and procedures.

9.1-5 What resources are available for training materials?

<797> lists the basic requirements. Didactic training[11] and a number of resources are available from ASHP. See **Exhibit 9-1**. CriticalPoint LLC[12] and other organizations provide hands-on training.

EXHIBIT 9-1. Sterile Compounding Resources Available from ASHP

Resource Center
- Sterile Compounding Resource Center at www.ashp.org

Guidelines
- Compounding Sterile Preparations
- Handling Hazardous Drugs
- Outsourcing Sterile Compounding Services
- Pharmacy-Prepared Ophthalmic Products

Publications
- *Aseptic Compounding Technique: Learning and Mastering the Ritual* (Jordan ZT, ASHP, 2018
- *Basics of Aseptic Compounding Technique Videos and Training*
- *Compounding Sterile Preparations*, 4th ed. (Buchanan EC, Forrey RA, Schneider PJ, ASHP, 2018)
- *Compounding Sterile Preparations: ASHP's Video Guide to Chapter <797>*
- *USP <800> Course*
- *Extended Stability for Parenteral Drugs*, 6th ed. (Dellamorte Bing C, Nowobilski-Vasilios A, ASHP, 2017)
- *Getting Started in Aseptic Compounding*
- *Hazardous Drugs—Handling in Healthcare Settings: ASHP's Guide to USP Chapter <800>*
- *The Chapter <800> Answer Book,* 2nd ed. (Kienle PC, ASHP, 2020)

9.1-6 If a pharmacist has BPS board certification, do they need additional training?

Yes. Though the Board of Pharmacy Specialties Certified Sterile Compounding Pharmacist (BCSCP) certification[13] indicates the ability to successfully complete the didactic material, they also must be able to demonstrate successful completion of the same competencies you require for any compounder and demonstrate knowledge of your organizational policies and procedures.

9.1-7 If a technician has technician certification, do they need additional training?

Yes. The Pharmacy Technician Certification Board (PTCB) certification of CPhT indicates the ability to successfully complete a general pharmacy technician examination; it is not specific to sterile compounding. PTCB also has an additional technician certification for compounding sterile preparations.[14] Any pharmacy technician who mixes CSPs must be able to demonstrate successful completion of the same competencies you require for any compounder and demonstrate knowledge of your organizational policies and procedures.

9.1-8 If a technician has both a CPhT and the additional sterile compounding certification, do they need additional training?

Yes. Though the additional sterile compounding certification from the Pharmacy Technician Certification Board (PTCB) of Certified Compounded Sterile Preparation Technician (CSPT™)[14] indicates the ability to successfully complete the didactic material, they also must be able to demonstrate successful completion of the same competencies you require for any compounder and demonstrate knowledge of your organizational policies and procedures.

9.1-9 Our clerkship students are trained by the college prior to coming to hospital sites. Do they need additional training?

Yes. They also must be able to demonstrate successful completion of the same competencies you require for any compounder and demonstrate knowledge of your organizational policies and procedures if they will be compounding sterile preparations at your organization. Even if they have a document indicating successful completion of the media fill and gloved fingertip and thumb testing at the college, it still must be repeated at your organization because those tests must reflect the facility conditions for your patients.

9.1-10 Who has to oversee the training and check off new personnel?

The oversight of this must be done by your designated person, but that person can delegate other qualified personnel to train and confirm competence of others.

9.1-11 Can a technician be the person who OKs a staff member's training, or does it have to be a pharmacist?

<797> does not restrict this to a pharmacist. Some states may require that this individual is a pharmacist.

9.1-12 Does training need to be documented?

Yes.

9.1-13 Does training documentation have to be written?

It can be written or electronic. Be sure it is retrievable because regulators and accreditation organization surveyors often ask to see these documents.

9.1-14 Do people who aren't compounding need training if they enter the IV room?

Yes. Anyone entering the sterile compounding suite or segregated compounding area (SCA) needs to be aware of restrictions. This includes administrative personnel, environmental services, surveyors, students, or anyone else. If they are not compounding or overseeing compounding, they don't necessarily need the same training as individuals who compound, but they still need to know what they may and may not do within the sterile compounding area.

9.1-15 If pharmacists just check IVs but don't compound, do they need training?

Yes. There is no "just checking" with compounding. Whoever is checking needs to be fully competent to perform compounding, so they know what they are checking. They need to complete all the required tests at the same frequency as any personnel who compound CSPs.

9.1-16 I'm the only pharmacist. Who has to train me?

A qualified person needs to train you. They could come to your site or you could attend an external program.

9.2 HAND HYGIENE

9.2-1 Is hand hygiene the same thing as hand washing?

Hand washing is a component of hand hygiene. See the CDC document on Hand Hygiene in Healthcare Setting[20] for complete information.

9.2-2 Where can I find a comprehensive description of hand hygiene?

See the CDC document on Hand Hygiene in Healthcare Settings[20] for complete information. The infection preventionist at your organization is a great source for this information.

9.2-3 Is soap and water OK to use for hand hygiene?

Yes. Hand washing with soap and water is required when compounding sterile preparations.

9.2-4 How often does a compounder need to demonstrate proper hand hygiene?

<797> requires proper hand hygiene to be documented initially, then at least every 6 months.

9.2-5 Do people who are just checking IVs need to show competence in hand hygiene?

Yes. There is no "just checking" with compounding. Whoever is checking needs to be fully competent to perform compounding, so they know what they are checking. They need to complete all the required tests at the same frequency as any personnel who compound CSPs.

9.3 GARBING

9.3-1 How often does a compounder need to demonstrate proper garbing?

<797> requires proper garbing to be documented initially, then at least every 6 months.

9.3-2 Do people who are just checking IVs need to demonstrate proper garbing procedures?

Yes. There is no "just checking" with compounding. Whoever is checking needs to be fully competent to perform compounding, so they know what they are checking. They need to complete all the required tests at the same frequency as any personnel who compound CSPs.

9.4 GLOVED FINGERTIP AND THUMB TEST

9.4-1 What is the purpose of the gloved fingertip and thumb test?

There are two purposes:

- The initial gloved fingertip and thumb test is done to demonstrate that compounders can repeatedly garb without contaminating themselves.
- The requalification gloved fingertip and thumb test is done after actual compounding to demonstrate the ability to maintain asepsis while compounding.

9.4-2 What type of media is used for a gloved fingertip and thumb test?

Use trypticase soy agar (TSA) that has been neutralized (e.g., with lecithin, polysorbate 80 [Tween 80]).

9.4-3 What is the proper procedure for doing a gloved fingertip and thumb test?

- Obtain one sampling device (e.g., plate) per hand.
- Label each sampling device with the compounder's name or initials, date and time of sampling, and right or left hand.
- Do NOT apply sterile 70% isopropyl alcohol or other solutions to the gloves immediately prior to sampling because this could cause false–negative results
- Sample each hand by rolling fingers and thumb over the surface of the agar.

9.4-4 Where are the samples kept?

The media devices need to be incubated. The incubator temperature must be monitored and within the defined range.

9.4-5 How are the samples incubated?

- Store the media during incubation so condensation will not drip onto the surface. For example, store a media plate upside down.

- Incubate the samples at 30–35°C for at least 48 hours then at 20–25°C for at least 5 more days.
- Record the number of colony-forming units (CFUs) per hand. Total the number of CFUs on six plates (for the initial test) or both plates (for the requalifying test).

9.4-6 How and where is the initial gloved fingertip and thumb test done?

The person needs to follow your procedures, completing the full hand hygiene and garbing required for sterile compounding. Sample the person's glove inside a classified area (e.g., the anteroom) or the SCA. This needs to be repeated three separate times.

9.4-7 Can a person garb once and use three sets of plates at one time for the initial gloved fingertip and thumb test?

No. The purpose is to demonstrate the ability to repeatedly garb aseptically. The full hand hygiene and garbing must be done three separate times.

9.4-8 Do the three separate garbing sessions need to be done on the same day?

No. They can be done on the same day or on separate days. Three successful gloved fingertip and thumb tests must be completed before being allowed to compound independently.

9.4-9 How and where is the requalification gloved fingertip and thumb test done?

Sample the compounder's gloves after completing a media fill test in the primary engineering control (PEC).

9.4-10 We use a compounding aseptic isolator (CAI). Does the gloved fingertip and thumb test need to be done inside the CAI?

Yes. The compounder needs to place sterile gloves over the gloves on the compounding isolator sleeves. The gloved fingertip and thumb test is done on those gloves. This applies to both the initial and the requalifying test, because it needs to reflect the garbing and gloving procedure used at your organization.

9.4-11 How often is the requalification gloved fingertip and thumb test required?

At least every 6 months.

9.4-12 Are three sets of media plates required for the requalification gloved fingertip and thumb test?

No. One set of plates—one plate for each hand—is required for the requalification gloved fingertip and thumb test.

9.4-13 If someone passes two of the initial three gloved fingertip and thumb tests, do they have to repeat all three or just one?

They need to repeat all three (a total of six plates).

9.4-14 Is the training gloved fingertip and thumb test different from the one for retraining?

The procedure is the same. The location is different; the initial test is done in the anteroom (if you have a cleanroom suite) or the SCA (if you have an SCA) and the requalification test is done in the PEC. The action levels are different.

9.4-15 What does the *action level* mean?

The action level is the limit of growth—identified as CFUs—allowed. If the number of CFUs exceed the action level, some type of procedure is necessary to identify the reason and correct it.

9.4-16 Do the action level numbers apply to one hand or both hands?

Both hands must be tested. The action levels are based on the total CFUs detected (right hand plus left hand).

9.4-17 Do you need to sample both hands?

Yes. The four fingers and thumb of each hand needs to be sampled on a separate plate.

9.4-18 Can one plate be used for both hands?

No. The four fingers and thumb of each hand needs to be sampled on a separate plate.

9.4-19 What is the action level for the initial gloved fingertip and thumb test?

The action level for the initial gloved fingertip and thumb test is anything greater than zero. This means that any CFUs detected on six plates (three tests of each hand) is unacceptable. The person needs to repeat the garbing and gloved fingertip and thumb test three times (for a total of six plates).

9.4-20 What is the action level for the requalification gloved fingertip and thumb test?

The action level for the requalification gloved fingertip and thumb test is anything greater than three. This means that any more than three CFUs detected on two plates (one test of each hand) is unacceptable. The person needs to repeat the test until it is acceptable.

9.4-21 Why must I have no growth on a gloved fingertip and thumb test when I'm learning, but when I'm really mixing IVs for patients, I can have some growth?

This seems counterintuitive, but it's not because the two tests are for different purposes.

The *initial gloved fingertip and thumb test* is done to demonstrate compounders can repeatedly garb without contaminating themselves. It's done under controlled training conditions prior to actual compounding, so no growth on the media plates is allowed.

The *requalification gloved fingertip and thumb test* is done after actual compounding to demonstrate the ability to maintain asepsis while compounding. It's done after a media fill test (which simulates the most complex CSP mixed) so is under conditions that reflect actual compounding.

9.4-22 If someone exceeds the action level, can they compound?

No. A new compounder needs to successfully complete the initial three gloved fingertip and thumb tests and a person who has already demonstrated competence to compound needs to successfully complete the requalification gloved fingertip and thumb test to compound.

9.4-23 Do nurses who only mix immediate-use CSPs need to do a gloved fingertip and thumb test?

Personnel who mix only immediate-use CSPs are not required by <797> to complete a gloved fingertip and thumb or media fill test.

9.4-24 Do the nuclear medicine technologists need to do a gloved fingertip and thumb test?

USP General Chapter <825> Radiopharmaceuticals—Preparation, Compounding, Dispensing, and Repackaging describes limitations of immediate use of sterile radiopharmaceuticals.

Note: This is a different definition than immediate use in <797>. Most hospital nuclear medicine department personnel only prepare sterile radiopharmaceuticals that meet the <825> immediate-use definition. If that is the case in your organization, the nuclear medicine technologists are not required to complete a gloved fingertip and thumb test by <825>. However, if more extensive compounding occurs in the nuclear medicine department, the gloved fingertip and thumb test and other requirements may need to be met. See <825> for full information. If the nuclear medicine technologists compound any sterile nonradiopharmaceuticals, they must comply with the requirements in <797>.

9.5 ASEPTIC TECHNIQUE

9.5-1 What is the definition of *aseptic technique*?

It is the process used to maintain asepsis during the compounding of sterile preparations. It encompasses proper garbing, maintenance of proper procedures, manipulations of components, and other procedural processes.

9.5-2 Is there a USP chapter about aseptic technique?

No, but refer to the information in ASHP's *Compounding Sterile Preparations*, 4th edition[26] and other compounding resources.

9.5-3 Does ASHP have any resources to teach aseptic technique?

Yes. There are a number of resources. See **Exhibit 9-1**. Remember that skills such as aseptic technique are best learned by reviewing didactic material, watching a skilled compounder, then providing return demonstration to the skilled compounder who can critique technique.

9.5-4 Is the aseptic technique nurses learn or the technique used in the operating room (OR) the same thing as the aseptic technique we need to use when compounding?

The principles are the same, but the procedures vary because the precision of sterile compounding differs from patient care activities.

9.5-5 What test is used to demonstrate competence in aseptic technique?

The media fill test simulates sterile compounding and is used to demonstrate the ability to aseptically manipulate the most complex CSP that a compounder could be expected to mix.

9.6 MEDIA FILL TEST

9.6-1 What is the purpose of the media fill test?

The media fill test simulates sterile compounding and is used to demonstrate the ability to aseptically manipulate the most complex CSP that a compounder could be expected to mix.

9.6-2 How often does a media fill test have to be done?

Every sterile compounder needs to successfully complete a media fill test initially and at least every 6 months.

9.6-3 How do I design a media fill test?

Determine the most complex CSP that a compounder at your site would need to mix. You need to simulate that. It may be the number of manipulations, the need to achieve sterility rather than only maintain sterility, use of specific equipment, or other factors that increase the complexity of the CSPs mixed at your site.

9.6-4 Can I use a commercially available kit for a media fill test?

Yes, if it mimics the most complex CSP you mix.

9.6-5 What kind of media and devices are used for a media fill test?

Soybean-casein digest media is used. Your laboratory can provide you with sources. The devices are dependent on the most complex CSP you mix. It may be IV bags and vials. It may be an automated compounder, ambulatory infusion pump, or other container or device. Mimic the components and devices you use.

9.6-6 We use a CAI. Do we still need to do a media fill test?

Yes. The media fill test is required for anyone who compounds CSPs in a Category 1 or 2 facility. (See Section 11.)

9.6-7 Does everyone on staff need to do the same media fill test?

Not necessarily, unless required by your state or organizational policy. However, consider your staffing patterns and work needs. The media fill test needs to mimic the most complex CSP a compounder would be asked to prepare.

9.6-8 What is the proper procedure for doing a media fill test?

The procedure is dependent on the media fill test you use. Commercially available kits have instructions that meet the components in the kit. If you create your own, develop a procedure that mimics the manipulations necessary to mix the most complex CSP you prepare.

9.6-9 If I mix nonsterile-to-sterile preparations, can I use purchased soybean-casein digest media?

If you mix nonsterile-to-sterile CSPs, you need to start with nonsterile soybean-casein digest powder.

9.6-10 Can I start with nonsterile media and mix it myself?

If you are simulating nonsterile-to-sterile preparations, you need to do that, and to include at least one positive control to show growth promotion capability. See the section in *USP General Chapter <71> Sterility Tests* that details Culture Media and Incubation Temperatures, Growth Promotion Test of Aerobes, Anaerobes, and Fungi.[27]

9.6-11 Is there specific information I need to keep concerning the media used?

You need to keep the lot-specific Certificate of Analysis (CoA) that says it will support the growth of microorganisms.

9.6-12 Do I need an incubator?

The tests need to be incubated. Pharmacy doesn't necessarily need to have the incubator in the department. Many organizations have the microbiology laboratory incubate the tests. If you do have an incubator, it cannot be inside the sterile compounding area.

9.6-13 Can I use a mannitol warmer to incubate the media fill tests?

No. Most mannitol warmers are not sufficiently controlled or calibrated to maintain the required incubation temperatures.

9.6-14 At what temperature and for how long do the media fill tests need to be incubated?

Incubate them for 7 days at 20–25°C, then for an additional 7 days at 30–35°C.

9.6-15 Is there an action level for media fill tests?

The media fill test is pass/fail. A negative test is good; no turbidity or color change is present after incubation. A failed test is one where turbidity or other growth occurs prior to the end of the 14-day incubation period.

9.6-16 Where is the initial media fill test done?

The media fill test simulates the most complex CSP you mix. It is done inside the PEC.

9.6-17 Where is the requalification media fill test done?

The media fill test simulates the most complex CSP you mix. It is done inside the PEC.

9.6-18 What should be documented?

Compounder's name, date of the test, media used (manufacturer, lot number, expiry), incubation location and temperature records, results of the test, who read the results, and who documented the results.

9.6-19 Do nurses who only mix immediate-use CSPs need to do a media fill test?

Personnel who mix only immediate-use CSPs are not required by <797> to complete a gloved fingertip or media fill test.

9.6-20 Do the nuclear medicine technologists need to do a media fill test?

<825> describes limitations of immediate use of sterile radiopharmaceuticals.

Note: This is a different definition than immediate use in <797>. Most hospital nuclear medicine department personnel only compound sterile radiopharmaceuticals that meet the <825> immediate-use definition. If that is the case in your organization, the nuclear medicine technologists are not required to complete a media fill test by <825>. However, if more extensive compounding occurs in the nuclear medicine department, the media fill test and other requirements may need to be met. See <825> for full information. If the nuclear medicine technologists compound any sterile nonradiopharmaceuticals, they must comply with the requirements in <797>.

9.7 REQUALIFICATION

9.7-1 How often does retraining need to occur?

Visual observation of hand hygiene and garbing and successful completion of gloved fingertip and thumb and media fills tests must occur at least every 6 months. Sterile compounders need to requalify concerning other core competencies at least every 12 months.

9.7-2 If someone has been on leave, or has not compounded for a while, do they need to demonstrate competence before they can compound?

If 6 months has elapsed since prior sterile compounding, they must requalify.

9.7-3 Do I need to document the requalification?

Yes.

9.7-4 Who needs to keep the records for training? Pharmacy? Human Resources? The individual?

The organization needs to maintain the documented competence in the employee's human resource records. It is up to the organization concerning the storage, but be sure that the records are retrievable because an inspector or surveyor could ask for them.

STERILE PRODUCTS AND SUPPLIES 10

(See Section 9 in USP <797>.)

10.1 GENERAL INFORMATION

10.1-1 What is the difference between the terms *products* and *preparations*?

Products are conventionally manufactured items. *Preparations* are compounded. Note that the FDA uses the term *products* for items compounded by an outsourcing facility.

10.1-2 What are conventionally manufactured products?

Conventionally manufactured products are those produced by pharmaceutical manufacturers. This differs from compounds, which can be provided by pharmacies (503A entities) or by FDA-registered outsourcing facilities (503B entities).

10.1-3 Does <797> deal with manufactured products? I thought it was only about compounded sterile preparations.

<797> is a comprehensive standard about sterile compounding. Conventionally manufactured products (e.g., intravenous [IV] bags, injection vials) are the key components of compounded sterile preparations (CSPs).

10.1-4 What are considered components of a CSP?

Components include the *ingredients* (i.e., drug, diluent, excipient), the *containers* (e.g., bags, syringes, vials) in which CSPs are placed, and the *closure-system* (e.g., cap) used.

10.2 USE OF NONSTERILE STARTING COMPONENTS

10.2-1 What is an API?

An API—active pharmaceutical ingredient—is defined by <797> as "any substance or mixture of substances intended to be used in the compounding of a preparation, thereby becoming the active ingredient in that preparation and furnishing pharmacological activity or other direct effect in the diagnosis, cure, mitigation, treatment, or prevention of disease in humans and animals or affecting the structure and function of the body."[3] It's informally referred to as *bulk powder* or *raw material*.

10.2-2 Do all components need to be marked *USP* or *NF*?

APIs must be obtained from a supplier that is registered with the FDA, so they will be marked *United States Pharmacopeia (USP)* or *National Formulary (NF)* if a monograph exists for the ingredient.

10.2-3 Why do I have to use an API that's from an FDA-registered supplier?

It's a federal regulation. Section 503A of the Federal Food, Drug, and Cosmetic Act requires bulk drug substances to be manufactured by an establishment registered with the FDA.[28]

10.2-4 I need to use an excipient that doesn't have a *USP* or *NF* monograph. Where do I get it?

Obtain it from an FDA-registered supplier if you can. If you can't, a designated person needs to ensure that it is of appropriate quality and suitable for use. See Section 9.3 in <797> concerning component selection.

10.2-5 How do I know the quality of the component?

You need a lot-specific Certificate of Analysis (CoA) for any component. That document tells you the quality standards and other information related to the component.

10.2-6 Is water a component?

Yes. Use *sterile water for injection* or *sterile water for irrigation* when mixing CSPs requiring water.[29]

10.2-7 I have some chemicals marked ACS. Are they OK to use?

Chemicals may be marked ACS (American Chemical Society), but that doesn't necessarily mean they are safe to use. They haven't been tested for pharmaceutical use in humans or animals.

10.2-8 I have a shelf full of old chemicals. Many are marked *USP* or *NF*. Are they OK to use?

If they are marked with an expiration date and that date has not yet passed, they are OK to use as long as the container and API appear undamaged. If they don't have an expiration date and you received them more than 1 year ago (or you can't tell when they were received), they need to be appropriately discarded.

10.2-9 If I received a chemical without an expiration date, do I need to assign a date?

Yes. Record the date of receipt, mark the date of receipt on the container, assign an expiration date that doesn't exceed 1 year, and mark the expiry on the container.

10.2-10 Can I start the 1-year expiry from the date I open the jar?

No. It has to be a maximum of 1 year from the date you received it.

10.2-11 The alum we use has a manufacturer's expiration date. Do I need to discard it after 1 year?

No. You can use the manufacturer-assigned expiry as long as you are confident that the ingredient, container, and closure (e.g., lid) are not compromised.

FACILITY DESIGN, ENGINEERING CONTROLS, AND EQUIPMENT

11

(See Sections 4, 5, and 21 in USP <797>.)

11.1 GENERAL FACILITY DESIGN INFORMATION

11.1-1 What are the minimum facility requirements for compounding sterile preparations?

CSPs must be compounded in an area that is specifically designated for sterile compounding and meets the requirements for Category 1 or Category 2 CSPs. The surfaces in the area need to be able to withstand the cleaning and sanitizing agents required following compounding. The floor cannot be carpeted. Temperature must be controlled to meet manufacturers' requirements for drug storage and for the comfort of personnel. Your state regulations may have additional requirements.

11.1-2 Are there different minimum facility requirements for compounding hazardous sterile preparations?

Yes. Hazardous drugs (HDs) must be compounded in a room that is separate from compounding of non-HDs. The room must have fixed walls, be negative pressure, be vented to the outside, and have the appropriate number of air changes per hour (ACPH). Sterile compounding anterooms and buffer rooms require at least 30 ACPH. See <800>[4] and *The Chapter <800> Answer Book*[8] for more information.

11.1-3 What engineering controls are required by <797>?

<797> requires a primary engineering control (PEC), commonly called a *hood*, and a secondary engineering control (SEC), the room in which the hood resides. (There is a special situation for compounding allergen extracts, which has a different requirement. See Section 11.14.)

11.1-4 Is an engineering control and a PEC the same thing?

A PEC, commonly called a *hood*, is a type of engineering control. The room in which the hood is placed is called an *SEC*.

11.1-5 What does *classified* mean?

Classified devices or rooms mean that they meet the requirements of the International Organization for Standardization (ISO) standard 14644-1 for classification of air cleanliness for cleanrooms and associated controlled environments, where the number of particles allowed is under the limit for that designation. PECs must be ISO 5 or better. (*Better* means fewer particles, which is a lower ISO number.) Buffer rooms must be ISO 7 or better. Anterooms must be ISO 7 or better if they open into a negative buffer room but can be ISO 8 (or better) if they open into only positive buffer rooms. Segregated compounding areas (SCAs) or containment segregated compounding areas (C-SCAs) are not required to be ISO classified.

11.1-6 Does the sterile compounding area need to be a separate room?

A cleanroom suite needs to have at least two separate rooms (anteroom and buffer room). An SCA should be a separate room but may be a separate area that is defined by a visible perimeter. A C-SCA must be a separate room.

11.1-7 Can noncompounding activities occur in the compounding area?

No.

11.1-8 Is it OK to use part of the intravenous (IV) room for office-related space, like order entry and processing?

No. Anterooms, buffer rooms, and SCAs need to be restricted to activities related to sterile compounding.

11.1-9 Is there a restriction concerning who can enter the IV room?

Only authorized personnel may enter the area, but that definition is up to you and needs to be described in your policies and procedures.

11.1-10 How much space is necessary for compounding?

That is based on your practice and needs. Be sure to allow space for any equipment you use for compounding. In many states, the state board of pharmacy regulations dictates a minimum area or linear square feet of counter space.

11.1-11 Can I use plastic curtains or drapes to define the compounding area?

No, not in cleanroom suites. <797> does not prohibit this in SCAs, but it's not a good idea. Dividers made of these materials are very difficult to keep clean. <800> required fixed walls, so plastic curtains or drapes are not allowed for a HD compounding area.

11.1-12 Does the hood need to be on emergency power?

<797> doesn't specify this, but some accreditation organizations standards do. In any case, it is a good idea.

11.1-13 Can I use the same compounding room for both nonhazardous and hazardous sterile compounding?

No. If you compound both nonhazardous and the National Institute for Occupational Safety and Health (NIOSH) Table 1 antineoplastic CSPs,[18] you need a separate room for each type of sterile compounding. Note that <800> allows you to entity-exempt some nonantineoplastic drugs on the NIOSH list of HDs if you perform an Assessment of Risk and identity and implement alternative strategies for containment and work practices. See <800>[4] and *The Chapter <800> Answer Book*[8] for details about hazardous compounding.

11.1-14 Do I need a separate room for receiving sterile products?

No. There is no requirement in <797> for receiving areas. However, do not allow totes or other external packages to be received or opened in your sterile compounding rooms; they have been in dirty areas and could contaminate your sterile compounding area.

11.1-15 What type of sink do I need, and where should it be placed?

Your sink needs to be easily accessible to your compounding area. Be sure your sink is big enough and deep enough so you can wash your hands and arms up to your elbows without splashing adjacent counters. Stainless steel is best; ceramic sinks are prone to chipping, so they become an infection control risk. Ideally, have a sink dedicated for compounding.

11.1-16 Should the sink be next to the hood?

Sinks are not permitted in the buffer room. The placement of the sink and the garbing practices you use need to be designed to work efficiently and safely together. Your sink needs to be at least 1 meter away from the hood in an SCA.

11.1-17 Why does a sink need to be at least 1 meter away from the hood?

It has to be at least 1 meter away from the hood to minimize the chance of microbial contamination from splashing.

11.1-18 Should the garb storage be adjacent to the sink?

No, but it needs to be close enough to efficiently garb. Placing garb right next to the sink could allow splashing and contamination of the garb.

11.1-19 Are there any temperature or humidity requirements for the sterile compounding area?

The temperature of the storage area for compounding components must be maintained based on the requirement of the CSPs or the components. Also consider the comfort of the compounders. <797> recommends a temperature not greater than 20° for the comfort of garbed compounders. <797> recommends a relative humidity below 60%.

Whatever temperature range and humidity is acceptable must be defined in your policies and must be monitored and recorded daily (when the pharmacy is open). It can be recorded on a log or by a continuous monitoring device; the information must be retrievable. Staff members need to know what to do if the temperature or humidity is out of range. Thermometers and humidity monitoring devices must be calibrated or verified at least every 12 months or as required by the manufacturer. Some regulators and accreditation organizations require calibration at least every 12 months.

11.1-20 If the humidity is low, should I put in a humidifier?

No. Don't add any water sources like this to the area. There is no need to adjust for low humidity in compounding areas.

11.1-21 What are the minimum air changes per hour required by <797>?

ISO 7 areas require at least 30 ACPH. ISO 8 areas required at least 20 ACPH.

Area	Minimum ACPH
Anteroom that opens only into a positive buffer room(s)	20
Anteroom that opens into any negative buffer room	30
Positive pressure buffer room	30
Negative pressure buffer room	30

Up to 15 ACPH may come from a PEC that is vented back into the room. At least 15 must come from the air handling system.

11.1-22 Can I depend on any type of PEC to be able to contribute 15 ACPH?

No. Laminar airflow workbenches (LAFWs), compounding aseptic isolators (CAIs), biological safety cabinets (BSCs), and containment ventilated enclosures (CVEs) that are vented into the room may contribute up to 15 APCH. Compounding aseptic containment isolators (CACIs) and BSCs that are externally vented cannot contribute to the ACPH total. Your certifier needs to indicate the source and total ACPH on your certification report.

11.1-23 Because <797> lists minimum number of ACPH, is there any need to use a higher number?

Yes. Don't design for the minimum, because you will see changes over time. The number of ACPH needed to maintain the environment depends on the number of people in the room and the activities performed. As the high efficiency particulate air (HEPA) filters in the ceiling age, they become less efficient and don't allow as much air to pass through them. If your room has 30 ACPH when new, you will see a decrease as the room is used.

11.1-24 How many ACPH are required for an SCA?

An SCA used for nonhazardous drugs does not have a required ACPH. A containment SCA used for HDs must have at least 12 ACPH.

11.1-25 Where should the gauges be for the temperature, humidity, and pressure?

There is no specific information in <797> but consider placing them outside the sterile compounding area. That way, you don't have to enter the room to read the information.

11.1-26 What kind of finishes do I need to use for floors, walls, and ceilings?

Surfaces of ceilings, walls, floors, fixtures, shelving, counters, and cabinets should be smooth, impervious, free from cracks and crevices, nonshedding, and cleanable.

11.1-27 What documents should my certifier reference on certification reports?

Your certifier needs to use the Controlled Environment Testing Association's (CETA) certification guide for sterile compounding facilities[30] or a document that provides the information required by <797>.

11.2 STORAGE AREAS

11.2-1 I have heard that cardboard isn't allowed in the compounding area. Is that true?

No shipping cartons, corrugated cardboard, or uncoated cardboard is allowed in a cleanroom suite or SCA. Most accreditation organizations expect the facility to do a risk assessment concerning placement of cardboard. If this applies to your organization, be sure to designate the compounding areas as clean areas and restrict external shipping containers and corrugated cardboard from the area.

11.2-2 Can shipping boxes be taken into the compounding area?

No. Accreditation organizations often require the organization to do a risk assessment for storage of cardboard. Because any compounding area should be designated as a clean area, no external shipping containers or corrugated cardboard should be allowed in the sterile compounding area.

11.2-3 IV bags and other supplies used for compounding come in cardboard boxes. What is the best way to store these?

When the supplies need to be moved into the compounding area, remove them from the cardboard outside the area and place them in labeled plastic bins. If the supplies were not protected by plastic, you may need to wipe them with a suitable agent prior to placement in the bins.

11.2-4 Do storage rooms require a specific ACPH?

<797> does not have a requirement for ACPH in storage areas. <800> has a requirement of 12 ACPH for HD storage areas.

11.2-5 Is it OK to store supplies on the floor?

No. Do not place components or other supplies directly on the floor.

11.3 PRIMARY ENGINEERING CONTROLS

11.3-1 What should I look for when buying a hood?

The PEC, commonly called a *hood* is a sophisticated engineering control used for sterile compounding. It is not the same as a fume hood, so that term should not be used to describe the device required for sterile compounding. A number of manufacturers make PECs designed for sterile compounding. All must maintain unidirectional flow of air and must meet ISO 5 requirements for air quality. See <797> for complete requirements.[3]

11.3-2 How often do hoods for sterile compounding have to be certified?

Upon commissioning (when you first use it), at least every 6 months, and whenever it is moved or serviced.

11.3-3 Is there an industry guidance for testing/certification of a hood?

Yes. CETA publishes certification guides.[30] The PEC needs to meet the minimum requirements of the applicable guide.

11.3-4 Is it OK to turn off the hood when we aren't using it?

No. The hood must remain powered on except for servicing or moving.

11.3-5 Can I use the same device for both nonhazardous and chemo sterile compounding?

If you compound both nonhazardous and NIOSH Table 1 antineoplastic CSPs, you need a separate device for each type of sterile compounding. (<800> allows occasional compounding of nonhazardous CSP in a BSC or CACI in a negative pressure buffer room or C-SCA, but because any component or CSP compounded in that space needs to be considered potentially contaminated and must be labeled with personal protective equipment precautions, it is not a practical process.) Note that <800> allows you to entity-exempt some nonantineoplastic drugs on the NIOSH list of HDs if you perform an Assessment of Risk and identity and implement alternative strategies for containment and work practices. See <800>[4] and *The Chapter <800> Answer Book*[8] for details about hazardous compounding.

11.3-6 Is a robot a PEC?

Yes, if it functions as a device in which CSPs are mixed. The robot needs to meet the definition of the specific type of PEC is it designed to be.

11.3-7 How many people can work in one hood?

It should be limited to one. Some organizations allow two people to work in 8-foot hoods, but there must be a clear division between the workspace. Consider the medication safety issues that can present if more than one person works in a hood. The Institute for Safe Medication Practices' (ISMP) *Guidelines for Safe Preparation of Compounded Sterile Preparations*[31] provides a review of safety considerations.

11.3-8 Does the pressure need to be documented every day for the space in the CAI?

<797> does not require that, but the manufacturer of your CAI or CACI may recommend it.

11.3-9 Are CAIs Category 1 or Category 2 CSPs?

CAIs are the primary control. The category distinction is based on the SEC (room) in which the CSPs are mixed.

11.3-10 Does a CAI need to be in a cleanroom suite?

It needs to be in a cleanroom suite to use Category 2 beyond-use dates (BUDs) or in an SCA to use Category 1 BUDs. See Section 15.

11.3-11 We have a system that includes a camera inside the hood. Is this OK?

Yes, as long as the PEC meets certification requirements under dynamic conditions.

11.3-12 We have a system that includes a scale inside the hood. Is this OK?

Yes, as long as the PEC meets certification requirements under dynamic conditions.

11.3-13 We have a system that includes a touchscreen monitor inside the hood. Is this OK?

Yes, as long as the PEC meets certification requirements under dynamic conditions.

11.4 SECONDARY ENGINEERING CONTROLS—GENERAL INFORMATION

11.4-1 What is a secondary engineering control (SEC)?

The SEC is the room in which CSPs are mixed. A cleanroom suite has an anteroom and at least one buffer room and can be used to prepare Category 2 CSPs. An SCA is a type of secondary engineering control that can only be used to prepare Category 1 CSPs.

11.4-2 Are modular rooms OK to have?

SCAs can be either stick built or modular. They have the same facility requirements.

11.4-3 What kind of things do I need to be sure our architects, facility department, and contractor need to consider when designing our IV room?

Your sterile compounding area needs to be designed to meet at least the minimum physical facility issues and needs to reflect your workflow. What works at one place may not be appropriate for another place.

Be sure to consider the following:

- The space you need for the scope of practice—Be sure to know the potential for future expansion plans when the hospital's patient mix changes significantly (either by volume or specific services).
- The number of people you generally have in each room—The ACPH are minimum requirements and often need to be higher when more than one person is in the room.
- The air handling system capacity—Most compliant sterile compounding areas have a dedicated air handler.
- Temperature and humidity requirements of the rooms
- The pressure requirements of the rooms (anteroom, positive pressure buffer room for nonhazardous CSPs, negative pressure room for antineoplastic CSPs)—If you have other sophisticated needs (e.g., gene therapy), be sure to design appropriate space.
- The surfaces and finishes of the floors, walls, and ceilings
- Placement and number of ceiling HEPA filters
- Installation of ports to allow your certifier to test the integrity of the ceiling HEPA filters
- Low air returns and exhausts
- Exhausts for negative pressure rooms
- Space for solutions and equipment used for cleaning
- PEC placement
- Placement of sink
- Placement of plumbed eye wash
- Placement and types of doors separating the rooms
- Use of flat, cleanable sprinkler heads
- Placement of shelving

As you develop designs of the room, consider taping off the room size and hood and other equipment placement and walking through the area to ensure the space is adequate for your workflow.

11.4-4 Do all surfaces have to be stainless steel?

No, but stainless steel is a good choice because it is durable and will withstand the decontamination and cleaning needed.

11.4-5 Is every sterile compounding room an SEC?

An SEC must meet the facility requirements listed in <797>.

11.4-6 Is an SEC positive or negative pressure, or can it be neutral pressure?

In a cleanroom suite, the anteroom must be positive to the adjacent space. A buffer room used for nonhazardous CSPs must be positive to the anteroom. A buffer room used for mixing antineoplastic NIOSH Table 1 CSPs[18] must be negative to the anteroom. An SCA can be neutral/normal pressure. A C-SCA must be negative to the adjacent space.

11.4-7 Is a chemo room an SEC?

Yes. NIOSH Table 1 antineoplastics ("chemo") need to be mixed in a room with at least these characteristics:

- Room with fixed walls that is separate from nonhazardous compounding
- Negative pressure between 0.010" to 0.030"
- Vented to the outside
- At least 12 ACPH for a C-SCA and at least 30 ACPH for a negative pressure buffer room

11.4-8 How big should an SEC be?

<797> does not define this; your state board may. It needs to be big enough to adequately handle the compounding you do.

11.4-9 Is it OK to use the SEC for order entry if it's related to sterile compounding?

No. The SEC should be restricted to the activities directly related to sterile compounding.

11.4-10 Can the SEC be used to store drugs, IV solutions, and supplies?

Yes, but it should not be the general storage area. Remember that all supplies need to be cleaned at least every month, so anything inside the anteroom or buffer room needs to be removed for monthly cleaning.

11.4-11 Can I put shelving in my sterile compounding area?

Yes, as long as the room meets certification requirements under dynamic conditions.

11.4-12 Can I put a refrigerator in my sterile compounding area?

Yes, as long as the room meets certification requirements under dynamic conditions. Pass-through refrigerators are not allowed in negative rooms. Refrigerators are environmental challenges and must be meticulously maintained.

11.4-13 Can I put a printer in my sterile compounding area?

Yes, as long as the room meets certification requirements under dynamic conditions.

11.4-14 How do I calculate room air change rates?

ACPHs are calculated by using the room volume (length × width × height) and dividing it into the cubic feet of air per minute. (ACPH = CFM × 60/room volume.)

11.4-15 Do the monitors for temperature, humidity, and pressure have to be inside the IV room?

No. If they are outside the sterile compounding room, they can be read without the need to enter the room.

11.4-16 What is the distinction between the dirty and clean side of an SEC?

The *dirty side* of the anteroom is where you enter it from the uncontrolled (not ISO-classified) area. The *clean side* is where final garbing occurs. The garbing functions that occur in either side needs to be dependent on the placement of your sink and needs to be defined in your policies and procedures. (See Section 9.3 on garbing.)

11.5 ANTEROOMS

11.5-1 What is an anteroom?

The anteroom is a transition room that is part of the sterile compounding suite. It is a room where garbing occurs. It needs to be marked with a line of demarcation that separates the dirty side (the side you walk into) from the clean side (where gowns and gloves are donned). In most facilities, the sink is on the clean side of the anteroom. The doors to the buffer rooms are on the clean side of the anteroom.

11.5-2 What are the physical requirements for an anteroom?

The anteroom needs to be a separate room, positive pressure (at least 0.020" more positive that the adjacent space that is not part of the cleanroom suite), with at least ISO 8 air quality (at least ISO 7 if it opens into any negative space), and have the appropriate finishes on the floors, walls, and ceilings.

11.5-3 Does every sterile compounding room need an anteroom?

Every sterile compounding suite requires an anteroom. An SCA, C-SCA, or allergenic extracts compounding area (AECA) do not necessarily have to have anterooms but do need space within the area to complete garbing.

11.5-4 Is an anteroom positive or negative pressure, or can it be neutral pressure?

An anteroom must be *positive* pressure. It is designed with positive pressure to control antimicrobial and other particle contamination from entering the compounding suite.

11.5-5 Because our chemo room is negative pressure, does the anteroom for that need to be negative pressure?

The anteroom is always *positive* pressure. That protects the compounding suite from contamination.

11.5-6 Is more than one anteroom required if we have a positive and a negative buffer room?

One anteroom can serve both negative and positive buffer rooms.

11.5-7 How big should an anteroom be?

<797> does not define this; your state board may. It needs to be big enough to adequately handle the garbing and hand hygiene activities for the compounding you do.

11.5-8 Is there a minimum square footage requirement?

<797> does not define this, but your state board may.

11.5-9 Is there a minimum square footage requirement based on the number of people in the room?

<797> does not define this, but your state board may.

11.5-10 Is it OK to use the anteroom for order entry if it's related to sterile compounding?

The anteroom should be restricted to the garbing and hand hygiene processes. The more activities that occur in the anteroom, the more risk of microbial and other contamination.

11.5-11 Can the anteroom have a pneumatic tube?

No. That would be a significant infection control risk.

11.5-12 Can the anteroom be used to store drugs, IV solutions, and supplies?

It can but limit the amount of stock. Remember that all shelving must be cleaned monthly. If you use the anteroom for general storage of sterile products and supplies, you need to remove them at least every month for cleaning.

11.5-13 Can the anteroom have shelves?

Yes, if necessary, to store the products and supplies you store in the area.

11.5-14 What is the distinction between the dirty and clean side of an anteroom?

The *dirty side* is the side you enter from. The *clean side* is the side closest to the entrances to the buffer rooms.

11.5-15 What is the line of demarcation in the anteroom?

The line of demarcation separates the area in which you enter (dirty side) from the area where final garbing takes place (clean side).

11.5-16 What is the distinction between a wet and dry anteroom?

Some facilities have a more structured process for garbing and have separate rooms in which garbing takes place. The *wet* anteroom contains the sink. The *dry* anteroom does not. This is not a required design but can be used to support more controlled garbing. It is similar to the process used in pharmaceutical manufacturing facilities.

11.5-17 Can the anteroom have a sink?

Yes. Most facilities have the sink on the clean side of the anteroom.

11.5-18 Does the anteroom have to have a sink?

A sink needs to be available for sterile compounding hand hygiene. Most facilities have the sink on the clean side of the anteroom, but some more structured designs have separate anterooms (wet and dry anterooms). All organizations need to design their policies and procedures to support the design of the area.

11.5-19 My SCA is ISO 7. Does it need an anteroom?

You need an anteroom with an attached buffer room for compounding Category 2 CSPs because those require a compounding suite. If you have an SCA or C-SCA, a separate anteroom is not required but you are limited to compounding only Category 1 CSPs with a maximum beyond-use time of 12 hours if stored at room temperature or 24 hours if stored under refrigeration.

11.5-20 If I put a CAI in the anteroom, is that considered a cleanroom suite?

No. To be a cleanroom suite, your PEC needs to be in a buffer room that is entered from a separate anteroom. In this scenario, you might consider the anteroom an SCA (if all requirements are met), but you would be limited to the short BUDs of a Category 1—12 hours room temperature or 24 hours refrigerated. The type of PEC doesn't matter; the situation is the same if the PEC is a LAFW or a CAI.

11.5-21 What kind of finishes should be used for the floor, walls, and ceiling of an anteroom?

The finishes of an anteroom are the same as a buffer room: they must be "smooth, impervious, free from cracks and crevices, and nonshedding."[3]

11.5-22 Is it OK to separate the sides of an anteroom by putting tape on the floor?

No. The tape will loosen over time and create a surface to attract particles and other contamination. Install a permanent line, such as using a different color flooring.

11.6 PRESTERILIZATION AREA FOR WEIGHING POWDERS

11.6-1 Where should powders be weighed for preparation of sterile CSPs?

For Category 2 CSPs, presterilization procedures, including weighing and mixing, must be performed in a PEC. For Category 2 CSPs, this must be performed in a room that is ISO 8 or cleaner. Unless this is done in a room separate from the anteroom or buffer room used for compounding CSPs, you need to weigh and handle powders only when no sterile compounding is occurring. The room must be able to maintain ISO Class 8 while the powder-weighing is occurring.

Ideally, you should have a separate room that contains a PEC dedicated for this purpose, such as a containment ventilated enclosure (CVE) (e.g., a powder containment hood). The weighing and mixing would occur there, and then transported in a closed container into the buffer room for filtration (when applicable), compounding, and packaging. Personnel must be garbed the same as when working in an ISO 5 PEC.

11.6-2 Do I need a separate area for weighing powders if I never mix CSPs from nonsterile ingredients?

No. Most organizations mix CSPs only from sterile components. If this is the case, there is no need for a separate weighing room.

11.7 CLEANROOM SUITES

11.7-1 What are the minimum room requirements for a cleanroom suite?

A compounding suite must minimally contain a positive pressure anteroom and at least one buffer room (positive pressure for nonhazardous drugs or negative pressure for HDs).

11.7-2 What does a cleanroom suite have that an SCA doesn't have?

An SCA is not required to have HEPA-filtered ceiling air nor is it required to be ISO classified.

11.7-3 I have a combined ante/buffer room. Is this a cleanroom suite?

No. A cleanroom suite must contain a minimum of two rooms: an anteroom and at least one buffer room. The combined ante/buffer room that was allowed in the 2008 version of <797> may still be used for compounding CSPs, but it is now defined as an SCA so limited to Category 1 CSPs with a short BUD.

11.7-4 What is the ISO requirement for a cleanroom suite?

The buffer rooms need to be at least ISO 7. The anteroom needs to be at least ISO 7 if it opens into any negative room and must be at least ISO 8 if it opens into only positive pressure buffer rooms.

11.7-5 Are ceiling HEPA filters required?

Yes. The air entering the cleanroom suite (both the anterooms and buffer rooms) must come from HEPA filters placed in the ceiling of the room.

11.7-6 I have HEPA filters in the ceiling and the air returns about a foot down from the ceiling. Is this OK?

Probably not. The air returns/exhausts should be low on the wall to allow the HEPA-filtered air to sweep throughout the room. If the air returns are not low on the walls, your certifier needs to do a smoke study of the room to demonstrate that air is not stagnating in any area.

11.7-7 Does a cleanroom suite require an isolator?

A cleanroom suite requires any acceptable PEC allowed by <797>: a laminar air flow system (e.g., LAFW, BSC), a restricted access barrier system (RABS) (e.g., CAI, CACI), or a pharmaceutical isolator. A RABS or pharmaceutical isolator can be used in a cleanroom suite, but it is not the only acceptable PEC.

11.7-8 I have a combined anteroom/buffer room that is ISO 7. I heard this is no longer allowed in new <797>. Is this true?

It can still be used, but it must meet the requirement of an SCA and is limited to compounding Category 1 CSPs with a short BUD.

11.7-9 Where does the sink need to be placed in a cleanroom suite?

Most organizations design their compounding area with the sink on the clean side of the anteroom. <797> allows other sink placement, but the garbing policies and procedures need to be designed to work with the sink placement.

11.7-10 Are there separate requirements for a cleanroom suite used for chemo?

Yes. The negative buffer room used for HDs must have 4 minimum criteria:

▶ Room with fixed walls that is separate from nonhazardous compounding

- Negative pressure between 0.010" to 0.030" negative to adjacent space
- Vented to the outside
- At least 30 ACPH (12 ACPH is acceptable in a C-SCA)

See <800>[4] and *The Chapter <800> Answer Book*[8] for more information.

11.7-11 Can the air conditioning be turned off in the cleanroom suite when it's not in use?

No.

11.7-12 Can the number of air changes per hour be lowered when the cleanroom suite is not in use?

No.

11.7-13 Are portable HEPA filters OK to use?

They cannot be the only source of HEPA-filtered air. The air handing system must provide the minimum number of ACPHs. If used, a portable HEPA filter needs to be certified as leak-free.

11.7-14 How many people can work in a cleanroom suite?

That is not defined in <797>. It is up to you to determine the appropriate workspace requirements.

11.8 SEGREGATED COMPOUNDING AREAS FOR NONHAZARDOUS CSPs

11.8-1 What are the minimum room requirements for an SCA?

An SCA is a type of secondary engineering control but does not have all the controls of a cleanroom suite. It needs to be an area that is dedicated to sterile compounding. A separate room is recommended but not required. A visible perimeter must be defined to establish the boundary of the SCA. It cannot have unsealed windows, doors that go to the outside, or next to areas that could compromise the environmental control. (Areas like warehouses, restrooms, or dietary service areas could cause contamination—either particles, microbial, or both—to flow into the SCA.)

11.8-2 What can be mixed in an SCA?

Nonhazardous CSPs can be mixed in an SCA. If your Assessment of Risk allows the entity-exemption of some Table 2 or 3 NIOSH HDs,[18] they can be mixed in an SCA as long as you have defined the alternative containment and/or work practices required.

11.8-3 Can all CSPs be mixed in an SCA?

No. NIOSH Table 1 antineoplastics[18] and other drugs your Assessment of Risk does not entity-exempt cannot be mixed in an SCA but can be mixed in a C-SCA.

11.8-4 What does a cleanroom suite have that an SCA doesn't have?

A cleanroom suite, in addition to other controls, has and anteroom and buffer room, HEPA-filtered ceiling air and is ISO classified.

11.8-5 What is the purpose of a perimeter around the hood?

The visible perimeter defines the boundaries of the SCA, which must be restricted to activities related to sterile compounding.

11.8-6 Where does the sink need to be placed in an SCA?

The sink cannot be within the perimeter of the boundaries of the SCA. It needs to be accessible but no closer than 1 meter to the PEC.

11.8-7 Are there separate requirements for an SCA used for chemo?

An SCA cannot be used for mixing NIOSH Table 1 antineoplastic CSPs.[18] Those must be mixed in a negative pressure buffer room of a cleanroom suite or in a C-SCA.

11.8-8 What is the ISO requirement for an SCA?

An SCA is not required to be ISO classified.

11.9 CONTAINMENT SEGREGATED COMPOUNDING AREAS FOR HAZARDOUS CSPs

11.9-1 What are the minimum room requirements for a C-SCA?

<800> defines the requirements for mixing hazardous drugs.[4] A C-SCA used for compounding hazardous drugs must have four minimum criteria:

- Room with fixed walls that is separate from nonhazardous compounding
- Negative pressure between 0.010" to 0.030" negative to adjacent space
- Vented to the outside
- At least 12 ACPH (30 ACPH is required for a negative pressure buffer room in a cleanroom suite.)

11.9-2 Can I use a C-SCA for mixing all CSPs—both hazardous and not?

Once drugs and supplies are exposed to the environment used for storage and compounding HDs, they would all need to be considered potentially contaminated with HD residue. You can have two areas: an SCA for nonhazardous drugs and a C-SCA for HDs.

11.9-3 What does a cleanroom suite have that a C-SCA doesn't have?

A cleanroom suite, in addition to other controls, has an anteroom and buffer room, HEPA-filtered ceiling air and is ISO classified.

11.9-4 Where does the sink need to be placed in a C-SCA?

The sink needs to be directly outside or inside the C-SCA but no closer than 1 meter to the C-PEC or entrance to any negative room.

11.9-5 What is the ISO requirement for a C-SCA?

An SCA is not required to be ISO classified.

11.10 PASS-THROUGH CHAMBERS

11.10-1 What is a pass-through?

It is a chamber—usually around 2 feet by 2 feet by 2 feet in size—that is placed between two rooms to allow supplies to be passed into an area and completed CSPs to be passed out.

11.10-2 What components make a pass-through cleanroom-compliant?

It needs to have sealed doors on both sides that aren't open at the same time. Interlocked doors are best, which prohibit both sides to be opened at the same time. It needs to be cleanable; stainless steel is best. A window allows you to see what's inside the chamber.

11.10-3 How big can a pass-through chamber be?

There is no restriction in <797> but use of a chamber (about 2 feet by 2 feet in size) minimizes the potential environmental challenges.

11.10-4 Can a pass-through go from unclassified space into a cleanroom?

Yes, but be sure to place it to minimize potential issues with contamination. HEPA-filtered pass-throughs are available and could be considered.

11.10-5 What testing is needed for a pass-through chamber?

Your certifier needs to include the pass-through testing in your initial and every 6-month certification to be sure the use of the pass-through under dynamic conditions does not compromise the air handling in the room. If you have a HEPA-filtered pass-through, your certifier needs to confirm that the HEPA-filters meet the manufacturer's requirements and document that using CETA[30] or equivalent criteria. Include surfaces in the pass-through in your environmental monitoring.

11.10-6 How can I tell if the pass-through is contributing to problems in the IV room?

Check several things:
- ▸ Is your staff following the policies you established to ensure appropriate use of the pass-through?
- ▸ Does your certification report show that the pass-through was included as part of your certification?
- ▸ Does your environmental monitoring show any microbial growth?

11.10-7 We have a window that slides open between the anteroom and buffer room. Is this a pass-through chamber?

No. It is unacceptable to use. Have it replaced with a solid wall or a cleanroom-compliant pass-through chamber.

11.10-8 Is a window OK in the pass-through chamber?

Yes, as long as it is cleanable and an integral part of the pass-through chamber. You want a window in each side; otherwise, you would not know if there was anything inside the chamber.

11.10-9 Does the pass-through chamber need to be HEPA-filtered?

It is not required by <797> but may be required by your state. Consider use of a HEPA-filtered pass-through if it enters into a negative area.

11.10-10 I have a HEPA-filtered pass-through. Can I turn off the HEPA filter when it's not in use?

Check the manufacturer's information and confirm the use with your certifier.

11.10-11 Do HEPA-filtered pass-throughs need to be ISO classified?

Yes. That's the point of having a HEPA-filtered pass-through.

11.10-12 How big are pass-through chambers?

Generally, they are about 2 feet by 2 feet by 2 feet in size.

11.10-13 Is it OK to pass supplies through a pass-through?

Yes. That's the point of a pass-through. Be sure your policies define how you want it used.

11.10-14 Our pass-through isn't interlocked, but we only allow opening one side at a time. Is this OK?

An interlocked chamber is not required by <797>, but it is the best way to ensure proper use. If you don't have a device that is interlocked, your policies define the specific requirements and you need to ensure your staff is using it correctly.

11.10-15 We have a pass-through that is interlocked, but I can feel air moving in from the other room. Is this OK?

No. There is something wrong. It may be that the chamber is not properly sealed.

11.10-16 Is a cart-sized pass-through OK to have?

<797> does not define the size, but a cart-sized pass-through can compromise the air flow in a cleanroom and is challenging for cleaning. If you use this, your facility needs to be designed to allow proper use.

11.10-17 Is a pass-through refrigerator OK to have?

It is not prohibited in <797> but is prohibited in <800> for use into negative pressure rooms. Consider the risks even in a nonhazardous area, because openings the size of the refrigerator doors will likely affect air flow in the room. It needs to be meticulously cleaned and included in environmental monitoring to ensure you are not compromising the environmental control.

11.11 REFRIGERATOR AND FREEZER PLACEMENT

11.11-1 Is it OK to have refrigerators or freezers in a sterile compounding area?

Yes, and their placement must be considered when designing or renovating the area. A wall air return needs to be placed near the spot where the compressor could contribute particles into the room. There are refrigerators on the market that have a solid-state design and don't have compressors. You might want to consider them because they don't contribute particles to the room. A refrigerator is required by <800> for storage of NIOSH Table 1 antineoplastics[18] in your negative pressure buffer room, C-SCA, or in a separate HD storage room.

11.11-2 What type of refrigerator is required?

The refrigerator should be medical grade. Consider use of a refrigerator that uses a solid-state design (without a compressor) because those do not contribute particles to the room.

11.11-3 What does a "low wall return" for a refrigerator mean?

The air return is low on the wall to capture particles generated by the refrigerator.

11.11-4 Is a pass-through refrigerator OK to have?

It is not prohibited in <797> but is prohibited in <800> for use into negative pressure rooms. Consider the risks even in a nonhazardous area because the size of the refrigerator doors will likely affect air flow in the room. It needs to be meticulously cleaned and included in environmental monitoring to ensure you are not compromising the environmental control.

11.12 OTHER COMPOUNDING AREA EQUIPMENT

11.12-1 What other kind of equipment is used for sterile compounding?

Equipment other than hoods includes repeater pumps, automated compounding devices, mixers, and many other devices depending on the scope of compounding. Some state regulations list specific articles that must be maintained.

11.12-2 How do I know that mechanical equipment is OK to use?

When equipment is received, be sure to follow the manufacturer's instructions for set-up, have biomechanical engineering (or a department with a similar function) ensure the correct operation, provide in-services to staff, and document competence of staff to properly operate the equipment.

11.12-3 How can I be sure the equipment is USP-compliant?

USP does not certify equipment; that needs to be done by your independent certifier.

11.12-4 Can I have a telephone in the sterile compounding area?

There is no restriction in <797> concerning the equipment you may have in your sterile compounding room. The key is that the room meets the certification criteria under dynamic condition. However, consider use of a hands-free intercom rather than a standard telephone. For medication safety reasons, some organizations only allow outgoing calls from the sterile compounding area, because incoming calls could interrupt compounding.

11.12-5 Can I have a printer in the sterile compounding area?

There is no restriction in <797> concerning the equipment you may have in your sterile compounding room. The key is that the room meets the certification criteria under dynamic conditions. However, review your processes to be sure you only have the minimum additional equipment needed.

11.12-6 We use a system that has a computer tablet in the hood. Is this OK?

There is no restriction in <797> concerning the equipment you may have in your sterile compounding hood or room. The key is that the room meets the certification criteria under dynamic condition. Because the equipment is in your PEC, include it in your environmental monitoring to be sure it isn't adversely impacting the state of control of the PEC.

11.12-7 Is it OK to have a warmer in the sterile compounding area?

Is it necessary for sterile compounding? Evaluate the need. If it must be inside the sterile compounding area, be sure it is not adversely impacting the state of control of your room.

11.12-8 Is it OK to have an incubator in the sterile compounding area?

No. You don't want anything in the room that contains growth media. If you have an incubator in the pharmacy, move it to an area outside the sterile compounding space.

11.12-9 Is there a requirement to calibrate the equipment?

Thermometers, humidity devices, pressure gauges, and any other monitoring equipment need to be calibrated or verified at least every 12 months or more frequently if recommended by the manufacturer of the equipment, any regulatory agency, your accreditation organization, or organizational policy. Your certifier needs to supply you with documentation of the equipment used during certification; this should be a part of your every 6-month report.

11.13 COMPOUNDING IMMEDIATE-USE CSPs IN AMBIENT AIR

11.13-1 What does *ambient air* mean?

Ambient air is a condition that doesn't meet the ISO classification and other requirements of PECs or SECs; for example, the area in a nursing unit or procedural area where immediate-use CSPs are prepared.

11.13-2 Why is it OK to mix CSPs outside of an IV room?

In critical care areas or procedural areas there is a need to mix sterile products for urgent patient use. <797> allows for this and for preparation per approved labeling of sterile preparations to adequately take care of patients. However, use of immediate-use preparation should not be used when appropriate facilities and personnel are available to mix the CSPs under the proper controlled conditions.

11.13-3 Is the OR considered ambient air?

Yes. The operating room (OR) is ambient air so limited to immediate use and preparation per approved labeling.

11.13-4 What minimum requirements should an area used for immediate-use preparations have?

The area needs to be clean, uncluttered, and functionally separate.

11.13-5 If IVs are mixed in ambient air, do those areas need to be included in environmental monitoring?

<797> does not require this. If used for trending, recognize that you will likely have growth because the room is not ISO-classified.

11.13-6 Is a doctor's office considered ambient air?

Yes. Except for the preparation of allergenic extracts, any clinic area without a PEC and SEC is ambient air and limited to immediate-use and preparation per approved labeling.

11.14 ALLERGENIC EXTRACTS COMPOUNDING AREA

11.14-1 Do allergen extracts have to be prepared in an IV room?

Ideally, allergen extracts will be prepared in a PEC within a cleanroom suite or SCA dedicated only to that type of preparation. However, because of the type of CSP (self-preserved) and need for patient care purposes (a longer BUD to allow for appropriate patient treatment), a special type of control is permitted: an allergenic extracts compounding area (AECA).

11.14-2 Do allergen extracts have to be prepared in an SCA?

Ideally, allergen extracts should be prepared in a PEC within a cleanroom suite or SCA dedicated only to that type of preparation. However, because of the type of CSP (preserved) and need for patient care purposes (a longer BUD to allow for appropriate patient treatment), a special type of control is permitted: an AECA.

11.14-3 The allergists at our health system want to comply with <797>. What choices do they have for facility design?

There are four choices:

1. A cleanroom suite dedicated to preparation of allergen extracts
2. An SCA dedicated to the preparation of allergen extracts
3. Use of a PEC
4. Use of an AECA

11.14-4 What is an AECA?

An AECA is a dedicated area, used to compound allergen extracts prescription sets, that is similar to the facility design for an SCA. A separate room is recommended but not required. A visible perimeter must be defined to establish the boundary of the AECA. It cannot have unsealed windows, have doors that go to the outside, or be next to areas that could compromise the environmental control. (Areas like warehouses, restrooms, or dietary service areas could cause contamination—either particles, microbial, or both—to flow into the AECA.) A sink needs to be accessible for hand hygiene but cannot be closer than 1 meter to the work surface of the AECA.

11.14-5 If a pharmacy prepares allergen extracts, does it need to be done in a regular IV room or is an AECA required?

It should not be done in your regular IV room because you would be introducing mold, pet dander, and other components of allergen extracts prescription sets into your IV room. An AECA is not the only option you have, but it is one option. Consider establishing a separate SCA containing a PEC and use it only for preparation of allergen extracts prescription sets. For the PEC, consider use of a BSC (which does not necessarily have to be externally vented for this purpose).

11.14-6 Does an AECA require a hood?

An AECA is an alternative to a hood.

11.14-7 When is it OK to use an AECA?

The only use of an AECA is for preparation of allergen extracts prescription sets.

11.14-8 Can only doctor's offices have an AECA?

<797> does not limit this to a prescriber's office. It can be used in a hospital, but consider use of a separate SCA with a PEC for more control of the area.

11.15 SEGREGATED RADIOPHARMACEUTICAL PROCESSING AREA

11.15-1 Can radiopharmaceuticals be mixed in the regular pharmacy IV room?

No. Radiopharmaceuticals can only be manipulated in an area defined in the organization's radioactive materials (RAM) license.

11.15-2 Can radiopharmaceuticals be mixed in the laboratory's BSC?

No. Radiopharmaceuticals can only be manipulated in an area defined in the organization's RAM license.

11.15-3 Does the nuclear medicine department need an IV room?

It depends on what they manipulate. Most nuclear medicine departments do not compound CSPs; they manipulate conventionally manufactured products (such as kits for the *in vivo* labeling of red blood cells with technetium Tc-99m) and dispense radiopharmaceuticals prepared by a contracted nuclear pharmacy. If their activities are limited to these functions, they do not necessarily require a PEC, ISO classified area, or a segregated radiopharmaceutical processing area (SRPA). If their activities are more complex than this, they need the appropriate facilities as defined in *USP General Chapter <825> Radiopharmaceuticals—Preparation, Compounding, Dispensing, and Repackaging.* See <825>[5] for full information.

11.15-4 Does the nuclear medicine department need a hood?

It depends on what they manipulate. Most nuclear medicine departments do not compound CSPs; they manipulate conventionally manufactured products (such as kits for the *in vivo* labeling of red blood cells with technetium Tc-99m) and dispense radiopharmaceuticals prepared by a contracted nuclear pharmacy. If their activities are limited to these functions, they do not necessarily require a PEC, ISO classified area, or an SRPA. If their activities are more complex than this, they need the appropriate facilities as defined in <825>. See <825>[5] for full information.

11.15-5 What is an SRPA?

An SRPA is a dedicated area limited to sterile radiopharmaceutical preparation, preparation with minor deviations, dispensing, and repackaging that is similar to the facility design for an SCA. A separate room is recommended but not required. A visible perimeter must be defined to establish the boundary of the SRPA. It cannot have unsealed windows, have doors that go to the outside, or be next to areas that could compromise the environmental control. (Areas like warehouses, restrooms, or dietary service areas could cause contamination—either particles, microbial, or both—to flow into the SRPA.) A sink needs to be accessible for hand hygiene but cannot be closer than 1 meter to the work surface of the SRPA. See <825>[5] for full information.

11.15-6 Does my nuclear medicine department require an SRPA?

It depends on what they manipulate. Most nuclear medicine departments do not compound CSPs; they manipulate conventionally manufactured products (such as kits for the *in vivo* labeling dispense radiopharmaceuticals prepared by a contracted nuclear pharmacy. If their activities are limited to these functions, they do not necessarily require a PEC, ISO classified area, or an SRPA. If their activities are more complex than this, they need the appropriate facilities as defined in <825>. See <825>[5] for full information.

DAILY NONVIABLE MONITORING 12

(See Sections 4, 5, 17, and 20 in USP <797>).

12.1 What monitoring is required to be done daily?

You need to be sure your sterile compounding area is always in a state of control identified by <797>, best practices, and your policies and procedures.

Minimum items that need to be documented at least daily include the following:

- Temperature in storage areas for sterile products below the maximum permitted in manufacturer's labeling, which is generally less than 25°C
- Temperature in the sterile compounding areas, which should be less than 20°C
- Proper temperature in refrigerators (between 2°C and 8°C), freezers (generally between −25°C and −10°C, but some drugs require different temperature), warmers (based on the drugs stored), and incubators (varies based on the requirement of the media)
- Relative humidity in the sterile compounding areas, which should be less than 60%
- Calibration of sterile compounding equipment (e.g., automated compounders, repeater pumps)
- Pressure differential
  - Anteroom needs to be at least 0.020″ water column (wc) greater than the adjacent room.
  - Positive pressure buffer room needs to be at least 0.020″ wc greater than the anteroom.
  - Negative pressure buffer room needs to be between 0.010″ and 0.030″ wc less than the anteroom.
  - C-SCA needs to be between 0.010″ and 0.030″ wc less than the adjacent room
  - Negative pressure storage rooms must be at least 0.010" negative to the surrounding nonhazardous rooms.
  - Other facility or equipment monitoring as required by manufacturer's recommendations, regulatory agencies, accreditation organizations, or your policies and procedures.

12.2 What's the difference between nonviable and viable monitoring?

Nonviable monitoring are other parameters such as temperature, humidity, pressure, and equipment elements. *Viable* monitoring is the environmental monitoring for microbial contamination.

12.3 What's the difference between certification and monitoring?

Certification is the process conducted at least every 6 months by a qualified individual who examines the primary engineering controls (PECs) and secondary engineering controls (SECs) to be sure they are within the proper specification. Certification is part of *monitoring*, but your monitoring program needs to include other viable and nonviable elements required by <797> and <800>.

12.4 What monitoring is the certifier required to do?

Certification includes the following:

- Airflow testing of your PEC and SEC
- HEPA filter integrity testing of your PEC and SEC
- Total particle count testing of your PEC and SEC
- Dynamic air flow testing of your PEC

They need to use the CETA[30] Certification Application Guide 003 for Sterile Compounding Facilities or a comparable document.

12.5 Our certifier also does the viable testing. Is this OK?

Yes, but viable testing is different from certification. See Section 18 concerning environmental monitoring (EM). EM can be done by you or by your certifier.

12.6 What should the temperature of the sterile compounding areas be?

It should be less than 20°C.

12.7 What do I need to do if it's too cold in the sterile compounding area?

Talk to your facilities personnel who need to adjust the temperature. There is no minimum temperature requirement in <797>.

12.8 What do I need to do if it's too warm in the sterile compounding area?

Define this in your policies and procedures. Consider rechecking the temperature in 1 hour. If it is still out of range, notify your facilities personnel concerning the excursion. Prolonged temperature above 20°C contributes a risk of microbial proliferation.

12.9 Do I need to monitor the temperature of storage areas outside the intravenous (IV) room?

Yes. This is a general pharmacy issue. The medications and supplies must be stored within the temperature range defined by the supplier. Most drugs cannot be stored above 25°C. Brief excursions are allowed. See *USP General Chapter <659> Packaging and Storage Requirements.*[32]

12.10 What should the humidity be in the sterile compounding area?

It should be under 60% relative humidity.

12.11 What should I do if the humidity is too low?

There is no minimum relative humidity requirement in <797>. The concern with sterile preparations is too *high* a humidity because it can contribute to microbial proliferation. A low humidity may be a personnel comfort issue, but it is not a risk to the CSPs.

12.12 My facilities department says the humidity has to be at least 20%. They want to add a humidifier. Is that OK?

No. You cannot add in water sources to the sterile compounding area. There are other departments in the health system where low humidity is a risk (such as a potential for fires in the surgical suite). A low humidity may be a personnel comfort issue, but it is not a risk to the CSPs.

12.13 What should I do if the humidity is too high?

It must be corrected. Relative humidity above 60% can contribute to microbial proliferation.

12.14 Can we use a dehumidifier to correct humidity that is too high?

No. The correction must be made in the air handling system.

12.15 What should I do if the pressure in my anteroom or positive pressure buffer room is too positive?

Talk with your certifier for the best answer. Often, the certifier, your facilities department, and an air balancer work together to adjust the pressure. Having too high a positive pressure is not a violation of <797> because it requires only a minimum positive pressure of 0.020" wc to adjacent rooms.

12.16 What should I do if the pressure in my negative pressure buffer room or C-SCA is too negative?

Talk with your certifier for the best answer. Often, the certifier, your facilities department, and an air balancer work together to adjust the pressure. This is a serious issue because negative pressure greater than 0.030" wc presents a risk of pulling contaminants into the negative room from adjacent areas (including ceilings). Other manifestations often include bacterial or fungal growth from those adjacent areas and difficulty in closing or opening doors. A pressure range between 0.010" and 0.030" negative to adjacent rooms is required by <800>.[4]

12.17 If temperature, humidity, or pressure is out of range, do I have to report this to someone?

Your state may require it. Your organizational policy may require it. In any case, be sure to document the values and correction.

12.18 How often does our automated compounding device (ACD) need to be tested?

The ACD needs to be checked and documented daily (when used) to be sure it is working properly. For preventive maintenance, follow the manufacturer's recommendations and include the device in your biomechanical engineering's (or similar department) roster of patient-related equipment.

12.19 How often does our repeater pump need to be tested?

The repeater pump needs to be checked and documented daily (when used) to be sure it is working properly. For preventive maintenance, follow the manufacturer's recommendations and include the device in your biomechanical engineering's (or similar department) roster of patient-related equipment.

CERTIFICATION OF ENGINEERING CONTROLS 13

(See Sections 5, 17, and 20 in USP <797>.)

13.1 What does *certification* mean? How is it different from the monitoring I have to do every day?

Certification is the process conducted by a qualified technician who evaluates the primary engineering controls (PECs) and secondary engineering controls (SECs) for compliance with key elements required by <797>.

13.2 What qualifications does a certifier need?

Many companies provide certification services. All need to use the criteria included in the CETA Certification Application Guides (CAGs)[30] or equivalent documents including airflow testing of the PEC and SEC, high efficiency particulate air (HEPA)-filter integrity testing of the PEC and SEC, total particle count testing of the PEC and SEC, and dynamic airflow smoke pattern testing of the PEC.

CETA has a board certification for certifiers who have completed didactic and practical testing concerning all aspects of sterile compounding facility requirements. The designation CNBT (CETA National Board of Testing) indicates that the certifier has successfully completed all the requirements of this distinction.

13.3 What is CETA?

CETA is the Controlled Environment Testing Association, which is the professional organization for the sterile compounding certification industry.

13.4 What are CETA CAGs?

CETA does not set standards; they use existing standards, such as <797> and <800>, and develop guidance documents that incorporate all of the required elements. CAGs are their certification guides, which include those for evaluating the different types of PECs and sterile compounding facilities.

13.5 What should my certification report include?

Your report should include all the elements in the applicable CETA CAGs that apply to your devices and facility, confirmation that it was done under dynamic operating conditions, and that calibrated equipment was used for the test. The certifier should indicate which devices and areas pass all requirements, which may need attention for future certification evaluations, and which fail to meet the requirements.

13.6 What does *dynamic conditions* mean?

Similar situations as occur during your normal operating conditions. For example, if three people are usually in the buffer room, three people need to be in the room during certification. If an ACD or a repeater pump is kept in your PEC, that pump needs to be in the PEC during the testing.

13.7 Can I compound while the certifier is working in the room?

No, but you can simulate compounding or perform other activities (e.g., media fill and gloved fingertip tests, transfer of materials) that would normally occur.

13.8 Does the certifier need access to the ceiling above the intravenous (IV) room?

They need some way to access the ceiling HEPA filters. That may mean removing some panels in the ceiling. Ideally, have ports installed to allow the certifier to test the integrity of the filters without the need to physically access the space above the ceiling.

13.9 Is there a way to test the ceiling HEPA filters without crawling in the ceiling?

You can add ports that allow the certifier to test the integrity of the filters without the need to physically access the space above the ceiling.

13.10 My hood failed certification. Can I use it?

No, not until it is fixed and recertified. If a PEC fails certification, it means that one or more of the key required elements were not met. Correct the deficiency and have the hood recertified.

13.11 My room failed certification. Can I use it?

Maybe. If the room failed certification but the PEC passed certification, you may be able to consider the area as a segregated compounding area until you are able to have the room fixed and recertified. However, evaluate the reason the room failed to make a decision that supports safe practices.

13.12 We use an ACD. Should we take it out of the hood when the certifier tests the hood?

No. It needs to be kept in the PEC during certification because that is your normal operating condition.

13.13 We use a repeater pump. Should we take it out of the hood when the certifier tests the hood?

No. It needs to be kept in the PEC during certification because that is your normal operating condition.

13.14   We use an IV software system that has equipment in the hood. Should we take it out of the hood when the certifier tests the hood?

No. It needs to be kept in the PEC during certification because that is your normal operating condition.

13.15   Should the certifier do our environmental monitoring?

They can, but that is a different process than certification. See Section 18.

13.16   If the power goes off in our hood or room, does it need to be recertified before we can use it again?

It depends on the specific situation. Detail this in your policies and procedures. If the power is off for a short period of time (e.g., 1 hour or less), perform a total cleaning of the PEC prior to resuming sterile compounding. If the power is off for an extended period of time (e.g., a weather situation that lasts several days), that could present significant risk of microbial proliferation. In that case, consider a total cleaning of the PEC and SEC and take environmental samples. Based on your policy—and in conjunction with your facilities personnel, infection control practitioner, and designated person overseeing sterile compounding—assess the need for recertification prior to resuming sterile compounding.

13.17   Our certifier says our chemo room is "too negative" and that it's OK now but won't be in the future. Is this correct?

If the room is more than 0.030" wc negative than adjacent space, it does not meet the requirements of <800>. The information concerning this has been published since February 2016, but <800> did not become official until December 1, 2019. Perhaps your certifier made this statement in the time between publication and when <800> became official.

13.18   Do we have to get our hoods and rooms certified before we use them?

Yes. The certifier needs to certify the PECs and SECs prior to use. You will see the term *commissioning* used, indicating an evaluation of the devices and facilities prior to first use.

13.19   When does a hood need to be certified?

It needs to be certified on commissioning (prior to first use), at least every 6 months, and whenever it is moved or serviced.

13.20   When does a room need to be certified?

It needs to be certified on commissioning (prior to first use), at least every 6 months, and whenever the configuration of the room is changed that could affect airflow or other quality issues.

13.21 Can my facilities department check my hood?

Unlikely, because you need an independent qualified certifier who uses the criteria in the CETA CAGs or equivalent document.

13.22 We have a powder hood in our negative pressure storage room. Does it need to be retested every 6 months or every year?

Because this is for nonsterile compounding, <795> applies.[2] <795> requires PECs used only for nonsterile compounding to be certified every 12 months. However, because your certifier will certify your PECs for sterile compounding every 6 months, consider including the PEC for nonsterile use every 6-month frequency as well.

COMPOUNDING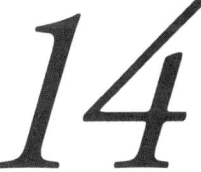

(See Sections 8, 10, 11, 12, 13, 15, 16, 19, 20, and 21 in USP <797>.)

14.1 GENERAL INFORMATION

14.1-1   How many people are allowed in the sterile compounding area?

That depends on your devices and facility. Anyone entering the sterile compounding area needs to be authorized to be in the area. Your policies and procedures need to define the routine and maximum number of personnel in each area. That information needs to be available to your certifier so he or she knows the number of personnel who need to be in the room during certification to identify the dynamic operating conditions.

14.1-2   Can students compound sterile preparations? If not, how can they learn?

Any personnel—employees or students—need to successfully complete training including media fill and gloved fingertip and thumb testing prior to independently compounding for patients. Some learning can be completed by observation and working with simulated conditions.

14.1-3   Are cellphones allowed in the sterile compounding areas?

No. Unnecessary items should not be allowed in the sterile compounding area. You need to define this in your policies and procedures. Consider the reason for needing a cell phone. It certainly would not be for making personal calls while compounding, so it is really needed?

14.1-4   Is it OK to play music in the sterile compounding area?

It is not recommended. Think of the medication safety issues—it could be a distraction.

14.1-5   Is mixing immediate-use compounded sterile preparations (CSPs) considered compounding?

It is compounding, but some of the requirements (such as media fill and gloved fingertip and thumb tests) are not required. It does not need to be done in a PEC or within a compounding suite or segregated compounding area. The area for immediate-use preparation needs to be clean, uncluttered, and functionally separate from other activities.

14.1-6 What special policies and procedures are needed for compounding intrathecal or epidural CSPs?

<797> does not distinguish among different sterile dosage forms. You need to address this in your policies and procedures.

14.1-7 Are vial tops sterile when they come from the manufacturer?

No. They are only dust covers. The septum of any vial needs to be appropriately disinfected prior to use.

14.1-8 Are there some drugs that I should not compound?

Yes. The Food and Drug Administration (FDA) has details on what can and cannot be compounded. State-licensed physicians and pharmacists that compound under section 503A of the Federal Food, Drug, and Cosmetic Act (FD&C Act) may only compound drug products using bulk drug substances that

- Comply with an applicable *United States Pharmacopeia (USP)* or *National Formulary (NF)* monograph if one exists
- Comply with <797> and <800>
- Are components of FDA-approved drug products if an applicable *USP* or *NF* monograph does not exist
- Appear on the FDA's list of bulk drug substances, which can be used in compounding (the 503A list[33]) if such a monograph does not exist and the substance is not a component of an FDA-approved drug product

In addition, bulk drug substances must be accompanied by a valid Certificate of Analysis (CoA) and must have been manufactured by an establishment registered with FDA under section 510 of the FD&C Act.

A pharmacist must not compound any commercially available product or any preparations that contain drug products on the FDA's *List of Drug Products That Have Been Withdrawn or Removed from the Market for Reasons of Safety or Effectiveness,* codified in Title 21 Code of Federal Regulations (CFR) 216.24.[34] However, a pharmacist may compound a commercially available product if, in the professional judgment of the prescriber, the product is modified to produce a significant difference between the compounded product for the patient and the comparable commercially available product.

14.1-9 Is the bulk list the same for pharmacies and for outsourcing facilities?

There are two separate lists: one for 503A pharmacies and one for 503B outsourcing facilities. 503B outsourcing facilities can only use bulk drug substances for agents that are in shortage or that appear on a list developed by the FDA for bulk drug substances for which there is a clinical need.

14.1-10 Is prepackaging medications into syringe containers considered compounding?

Yes. See *USP General Chapter <1178> Good Repackaging Practices*[35] and the FDA guidance documents concerning repackaging.[7]

14.1-11 Does ASHP have guidelines dealing with sterile compounding?

Yes. See the *ASHP Guidelines on Compounding Sterile Preparations*[36] and *Guidelines on Handling Hazardous Drugs.*[37] Some of the documents predate <797> so the USP standard needs to be followed when it is more stringent than the information in the ASHP document.

14.1-12 Are premixed solutions that I can buy from manufacturers considered compounded?

No. Items from a manufacturer are *products*, not compounded preparations.

14.1-13 Are premixed solutions that I can buy from an outsourcing facility considered compounded?

Yes. They are compounds. However, these items from 503B outsourcing facilities are called *products* (not preparations) in some FDA documents.

14.1-14 Is reconstituting a system like an ADD-Vantage™, MINI-BAG Plus, VIAL-MATE, or addEASE® considered compounding?

No, as long as you are attaching and activating these proprietary bag and vial systems for immediate administration. If you are docking the systems for future activation and administration, it is considered compounding, but you can use the beyond-use dates (BUDs) established by the manufacturer.

14.1-15 If I crush tablets or open capsules to make a CSP, is that an active pharmaceutical ingredient (API)?

No. Crushing, splitting, opening, or otherwise manipulating an FDA-approved drug does not create an API, the raw chemical that is used to produce the FDA-approved drug.

14.1-16 Is there an algorithm I can use to determine if it's appropriate to compound?

Consider this:

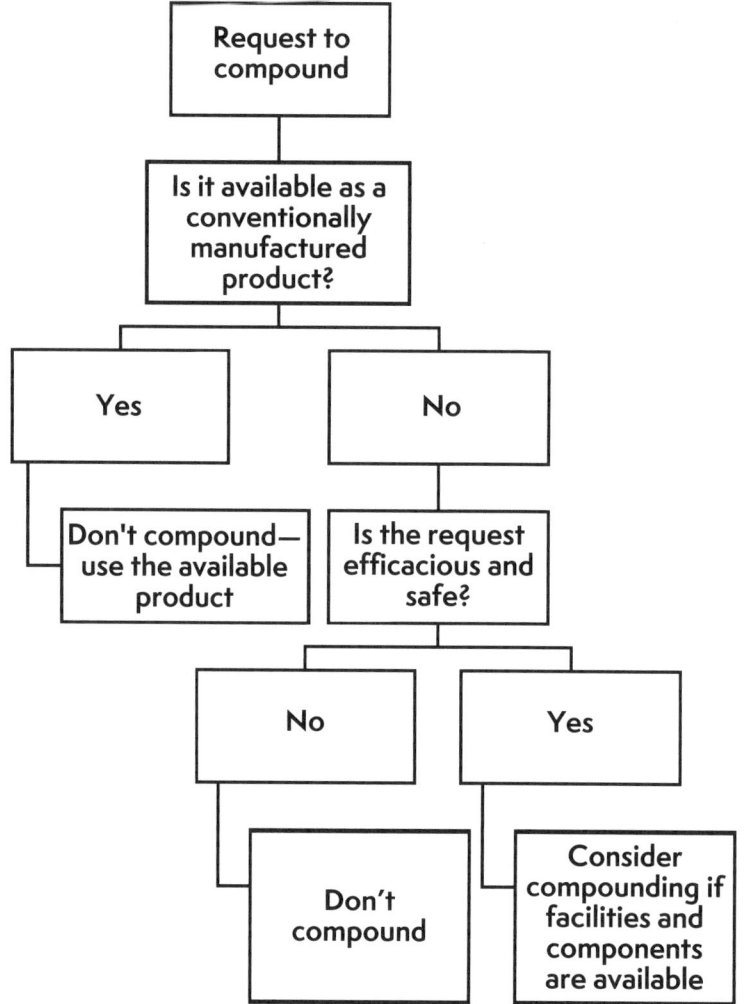

14.2 NONSTERILE-TO-STERILE COMPOUNDING

14.2-1 How do I know if an ingredient is nonsterile?

Sterile components are those conventionally manufactured products that are intended for parenteral use. They are marked as sterile on the final container. Anything else is not sterile. This includes APIs from suppliers, drugs not intended for parenteral use, and containers and closures that are not sterile.

14.2-2 Do I need a Certificate of Analysis for every ingredient in a compound?

All APIs used must have a lot-specific Certificate of Analysis (CoA). FDA-approved drugs do not need a CoA. Ingredients other than APIs or FDA-approved drugs should have a CoA.

14.2-3 How are CSPs that start with nonsterile components sterilized?

Ideally, they are terminally sterilized using steam (an autoclave), dry heat (an oven), or irradiation. If terminal sterilization cannot be done, they can be filtered. Note that filtration is *not* considered terminal sterilization.

14.2-4 What is the difference between terminal sterilization and filtration?

Terminal sterilization achieves a low probability of a nonsterile unit (PNSU). *Filtered* items that do not have the same assurance for this.

14.2-5 What is a bubble point test?

The bubble point test is a test of the filter that has been used to prepare a nonsterile-to-sterile CSP. You need to test every filter used for sterile compounding to be sure the integrity of the filter was not compromised during compounding.

14.2-6 Do containers need to be sterile?

Yes. All components of a CSP need to be sterile, including the containers and closures.

14.2-7 Is it OK to use an amber dropper bottle for sterile CSPs?

A standard dropper bottle is *not* sterile. You can obtain appropriate sterile containers and closures from several pharmacy suppliers.

14.2-8 If I batch 50 cefazolin syringes, do I need to do sterility tests?

If you are preparing CSPs from all sterile starting components and assigning a beyond-use date that does not exceed 4 days room temperature, 10 days refrigerated, or 45 days frozen and all the components are stable for that length of time, you do not necessarily need to perform sterility testing.

14.2-9 Are there additional requirements when working with blood components?

Blood components include platelet, red cells, white cells, autologous serum, etc. This is different from a commercially available blood product like albumin or intravenous immunoglobulin (IVIG). If you are compounding with blood components, you need to separate those activities from other compounding activities and develop and implement specific policies and procedures to avoid cross-contamination. See the Centers for Disease Control and Prevention (CDC) Biosafety in Microbiological and Biomedical Laboratories (BMBL) document[38] for additional information.

14.2-10 Are there additional requirements when working with albumin, IVIG, vaccines, or other biologics?

Compounding with biologics introduces additional risk into sterile compounding. For these commercially manufactured products, use the manufacture's information, which likely includes must shorter BUDs than conventionally manufactured products.

14.2-11 Are there additional requirements when working with radiopharmaceuticals like UltraTag™?

Yes. See *USP General Chapter <825> Radiopharmaceuticals—Preparation, Compounding, Dispensing, and Repackaging.*[5]

14.3 MASTER FORMULATION RECORDS

14.3-1 What is a master formulation record?

A master formulation record (MFR) is the recipe for a CSP. It allows a CSP to be reproduced with the same formula on repeated occasions.

14.3-2 When is an MFR needed?

An MFR is required for CSPs mixed for more than one patient and for all CSPs mixed with any nonsterile ingredient.

14.3-3 What needs to be recorded in an MFR?

<799> has a specific list of required elements:

- Name, strength or activity, and dosage form of all ingredients
- Type and size of the container-closure systems
- Complete instructions for preparing the CSP, including equipment, supplies, a description of the compounding steps, and any special precautions
- Physical description of the final CSP
- BUD and storage requirements
- Reference source to support the stability of the CSP
- Quality control procedures, such as pH testing and filter integrity testing
- Other information needed to describe the compounding process and ensure repeatability (e.g., adjusting pH and tonicity, sterilization method.

14.3-4 Is there a template form I can use to create an MFR?

See **Exhibit 14-1**.

14.3-5 We have a file with recipes for compounds. Is this the same as an MFR?

Yes, but be sure you have all the elements listed as required by <797>. An update of the recipes will probably be needed.

14.3-6 Where are sources of compounds available?

USP has over 150 compounding monographs. Some of these are sterile compounds. They are available in the *USP Compounding Compendium.*[1] The *International Journal of Pharmaceutical Compounding*[39] prints formulas in each edition of the journal. Other peer-reviewed sources can also be used.

14.3-7 If I make two different strengths of a CSP, do I need one or two MFRs?

Two. You need a distinct MFR for each unique compound.

14.3-8 Do I need to make an MFR for a one-time order or prescription?

This is not required by <797>, but it's a good idea to do.

14.3-9 Can I combine the MFR with a compounding record?

Yes. The MFR and the compounding record (CR) can either be separate or combined documents.

14.3-10 Is it OK to double or halve the listing on the MFR?

It depends if it changes any of the other elements. Your CR needs to note the quantity compounded.

14.3-11 Do the MFRs have to be printed out?

They have to be retrievable. They can be printed or electronic.

14.3-12 What happens if a change has to be made in an MFR?

Then it's a unique compound, so would require a separate MFR.

14.3-13 When changes are necessary, who can make them?

The designated person needs to be responsible for changes in an MFR.

14.3-14 Do I need an MFR for every antibiotic CSP I make?

If you will make it for more than one patient or if it includes any nonsterile component, you need an MFR. For example, many hospitals make 10 or more common antibiotic mixtures daily. Establish a separate MFR for each of these.

14.3-15 Does the MFR need to be in a specific format?

No, but it needs to include all the required elements.

14.4 COMPOUNDING RECORDS

14.4-1 What is a compounding record?

A compounding record (CR) is a record of the ingredients used to make a CSP.

14.4-2 When is a CR needed?

A CR is required for all CSPs.

14.4-3 What needs to be recorded in a CR?

<797> has a specific list of required elements:

- Name, strength or activity, and dosage form of the CSP
- Date and time of preparation
- Assigned internal lot number (e.g., prescription, order, or lot number)
- A method to identify the individuals involved in the compounding process and verifying the final CSP
- Name, vendor or manufacturer, lot number, and expiration date of each component for CSPs prepared for more than one patient and for any CSP prepared from nonsterile ingredients
- Weight or volume of each component
- Strength or activity of each component
- Total quantity compounded
- Assigned BUD and storage requirements
- Results of quality control (QC) procedures (e.g., visual inspection, filter integrity testing, pH testing)

If applicable, the CR must also include the following:

- Master formulation record reference for the CSP
- Calculations made to determine and verify quantities and/or concentrations of components

14.4-4 I've always recorded the information above for batches, but not for "one offs"—a single bag or two for one patient for a specific order. Do I need a CR for those?

You have to have a way to identify the specifics listed. <797> allows you to handle the single order CRs differently than batches, as long as you have a way to trace the information. Detail this in your policies. Some organizations run a duplicate label and maintain it but consider the potential patient safety issues with that process. Some systems create production labels that can be used. Others use camera technology. Your state may also specify maintaining this information for every CSP—including individual IVs—so be sure to follow that if it is more strict than the <797> requirements.

14.4-5 Do I have to record manufacturer's lot numbers for every CSP?

You have to record it for all CSPs made for more than one patient or any CSP made from nonsterile ingredients. You have to have a way of identifying the lot number of the component used for other CSPs, and that needs to be detailed in your policies and procedures.

14.4-6 Is there a template form I can use to create a CR?

See **Exhibit 14-2**.

14.4-7 Do the CRs have to be printed out?

They have to be retrievable. They can be printed or electronic.

14.5 ALLERGENIC EXTRACTS

14.5-1 How are allergenic extracts compounded?

The compounding process is no different from those used for other types of CSPs. The difference is the facility design allowed (see Section 11.14) and the BUDs permitted for the prescription sets compounded. See Section 21 in <797>[3], which details the information.

14.6 RADIOPHARMACEUTICALS

14.6-1 How are radiopharmaceuticals compounded?

The compounding process is no different from those used for other types of CSPs. The difference is the personnel protection that must be employed to minimize risk of exposure to radioactivity. See <825>[5], which details the information concerning facility design, personnel protection, and other details.

14.6-2 Is there a difference between what an outside nuclear pharmacy compounds and what is compounded in the hospital's nuclear medicine department?

That is likely. Very few hospitals have nuclear pharmacists, and those pharmacists generally work in the imaging department. Even fewer hospitals have a separately permitted nuclear pharmacy. Almost all health systems outsource their nuclear pharmacy services to an outside nuclear pharmacy.

The nuclear pharmacies prepare, compound, dispense, and repackage radiopharmaceutical based on Nuclear Regulatory Commission (NRC) requirements, state requirements, USP chapters, and precise policies and procedures. They provide patient-specific doses to your nuclear medicine department. The nuclear pharmacies comply with <825>[5] for radiopharmaceuticals and <795>[2] and <797>[3] for nonsterile and sterile nonradiopharmaceuticals. They may also have an SRPA for other radiopharmaceutials they manipulate.

Your nuclear medicine department likely administers those doses and may manipulate some commercially available products, such as those for the *in vivo* labeling red blood cells with technetium Tc99-m. Based on the complexity of the radiopharmaceutical manipulated, your nuclear medicine department may only need the facilities for immediate-use radiopharmaceuticals. Work with your nuclear medicine department to be sure your health system is in compliance with the appropriate sections of <825>.

EXHIBIT 14-1. Example Master Formulation Record for CSPs

NAME OF PREPARATION (name, strength/activity, dosage form) ☐ USP monograph ☐ Assigned name
INGREDIENTS (name, strength/activity, quantity/amount)
CALCULATIONS ☐ Not applicable
EQUIPMENT
COMPATIBILITY AND STABILITY INFORMATION (including references, if available) ☐ Not applicable
MIXING AND PREPARATION INSTRUCTIONS (Include order and duration of mixing, temperature/other environmental controls, etc.)
CONTAINER AND CLOSURE TYPE (Note both storage and dispensing containers, if different.)
BUD ASSIGNED ☐ 12 hours ☐ 24 hours ☐ 4 days ☐ 10 days ☐ 45 days ☐ BUD assignment based on: _____ ☐ Other reference (list reference and note BUD): _____
PACKAGING/STORAGE REQUIREMENTS: ☐ Refrigerate ☐ Protect from light ☐
DESCRIPTION OF FINAL PREPARATION
SAMPLE LABEL
QUALITY CONTROL PROCEDURES AND EXPECTED RESULTS

BUD = beyond-use date.

EXHIBIT 14-2. Example Compounding Record for CSPs

PREPARATION (name, strength/activity, dosage form):			Master Formulation Record	
CALCULATIONS:				
INGREDIENT (name, strength/ activity, dosage form)	AMOUNT (mL, g, etc.)	MFR	EXP DATE	LOT NUMBER
DATE AND TIME PREPARED:	Affix Label Here			
CONTROL/RX/ORDER NUMBER:				
TOTAL QUANTITY COMPOUNDED:				
PHYSICAL DESCRIPTION:				
BEYOND-USE DATE:				
QUALITY CONTROL RESULTS (if applicable):				
Prepared by:	Checked by:			

EXP = expiration, MFR = manufacturer.

BEYOND-USE DATES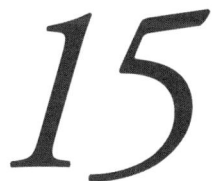

(See Sections 14, 15, and 16 in USP <797>.)

15.1 GENERAL BEYOND-USE DATE INFORMATION

15.1-1   Is a beyond-use date the same thing as an expiration date?

No. Manufacturers establish expiration dates for their products based on studies of the physical and chemical stability of their products, packaged in the dosage form marketed, when stored based on the requirements of the labeling. The beyond-use dates (BUDs) that compounders assign to preparations are much shorter because the validated testing is not done.

15.1-2   What's the difference among an expiration date, beyond-use date, in-use time, and infusion time?

All of these relate to expiry of products or preparations, but there are differences.

- An *expiration date* is set by the manufacturer based on scientific studies at specific storage temperatures.
- A *beyond-use date* is set by a compounder. It is shorter than the expiration date because the controls of a manufactured product are not available nor are studies done that support extended dating.
- *In-use time* is the time from when a product or preparation is opened or punctured until the point is can no longer be used.
- *Infusion time* is the time a product or preparation is being administered to a patient.

15.1-3   What factors go into the determination of a BUD?

Determining a BUD depends on several factors:

- Stability of the components—Including drugs, diluents, containers, and closure system
- Facility in which the compounded sterile preparation (CSP) is mixed—Category 2 in a cleanroom suite, or Category 1 in an segregated compounding area (SCA)
- Starting ingredients—All sterile or at least one nonsterile component
- Type of preparation—Aseptically prepared (including filtration) or terminally sterilized (autoclaved, use of dry heat over, or irradiation)
- Storage temperature—Room temperature, refrigerated, or frozen
- Use of a USP monograph

15.1-4 We have a cleanroom suite and mix CSPs from commercially available sterile products. What is the maximum BUD we can use?

The BUD always needs to be the shorter of the stability of the CSP components (drugs, diluents, container, and closure system) and the maximum allowable BUD listed in <797>.

In this scenario, the maximum BUDs depend on the storage temperature, so you will use following for mixing:

- 4 days or less for CSPs that will be stored at room temperature
- 10 days or less for CSPs that will be stored under refrigeration
- 45 days or less for CSPs that will be stored frozen

15.1-5 We make all CSPs in an SCA. What is the maximum BUD we can use?

The BUD always needs to be the shorter of the stability of the CSP components (drugs, diluents, container, and closure system) and the maximum allowable BUD listed in <797>. Because an SCA doesn't have all the controls of a cleanroom suite, you are limited to short BUDs:

- 12 hours or less for CSPs stored at room temperature
- 24 hours or less for CSPs stored under refrigeration

15.1-6 We make all our chemos in a containment segregated compounding area (C-SCA). What is the maximum BUD we can use?

The BUD always needs to be the shorter of the stability of the CSP components (drugs, diluents, container, and closure system) and the maximum allowable BUD listed in <797>. BUDs are determined by compliance with <797>. Maximum BUDs for CSPs mixed in a C-SCA are the same as those mixed in an SCA:

- 12 hours or less for CSPs stored at room temperature
- 24 hours or less for CSPs stored under refrigeration

15.1-7 We have a cleanroom suite and occasionally mix CSPs from nonsterile starting ingredients. What is the maximum BUD we can use?

The BUD always needs to be the shorter of the stability of the CSP components (drugs, diluents, container, and closure system) and the maximum allowable BUD listed in <797>. In this scenario, the maximum BUDs in the absence of performing a sterility test depend on the storage temperature, so you will use following for mixing:

- 1 day or less for CSPs that will be stored at room temperature
- 4 days or less for CSPs that will be stored under refrigeration
- 45 days or less for CSPs that will be stored frozen

15.1-8 Can we mix CSPs from nonsterile ingredients in an SCA?

Yes, but it is limited to a very short BUD: 12 hours for CSPs stored at room temperature or 24 hours for CSPs stored under refrigeration. Not all dosage forms can be appropriately mixed in an SCA.

15.1-9 We filter some CSPs mixed from nonsterile ingredients. Do we use the information about aseptically prepared or terminally sterilized CSPs listed in <797>?

You need to use the aseptically prepared information. Filtration is not a terminal sterilization process.

15.1-10 What is a USP monograph?

USP has some sterile compounding monographs available in the *United States Pharmacopeia–National Formulary (USP–NF)* or *USP Compounding Compendium*.[1] They are compounds that have undergone testing and may have BUDs that are longer than the charts in <797>. To use the BUD, you must make the preparation as directed in the monograph, use the same packaging, and use the same storage temperature.

15.1-11 Where can I find a USP monograph?

They are part of the *USP–NF* and also in the *USP Compounding Compendium*,[1] available at www.usp.org.

15.1-12 If we use a USP monograph, can we use the BUD listed in the monograph?

If you mix it with the specified ingredients and follow the monograph exactly (including final testing, if required), you can use the BUD in the USP monograph. Be sure to use the most current version of the monograph.

15.1-13 Can I use a USP monograph and extend the BUD beyond what's listed in the monograph?

No.

15.1-14 Can I use BUDs longer than those listed in <797> if I have peer-reviewed information that states a longer BUD?

No. The only way a BUD longer than that listed in <797> can be used is if a USP monograph is precisely followed.

15.1-15 If a drug's stability information is less than the BUD in <797>, can I still use the <797> BUD?

No. The BUD is *always* the shorter of the stability of the mixture or the allowed BUD times listed in <797>.

15.1-16 What are the required temperature ranges for room temperature, refrigerated, and frozen CSPs?

<659>[32] defines the temperatures:

▸ Controlled room temperature storage is between 20°C and 25°C.

- Refrigerated storage is between 2°C and 8°C.
- Frozen storage is between −25°C and −10°C.

15.1-17 Are temperatures listed in <797> in Celsius or Fahrenheit?

All temperatures are listed in Celsius.

15.1-18 Does the BUD include the time the drug is infused?

No. The BUDs start when the compounding starts and ends when the CSP starts to be administered to the patient.

15.1-19 How do I know how long a CSP will be infused?

You need to know the rate of infusion so you can appropriately mix the CSP. You need to develop an organizational policy on infusion time (which is often called *hang time*). Resources for information concerning infusion time are available from Centers for Disease Control and Prevention (CDC) in their document on Guidelines for the Prevention of Intravascular Catheter-Related Infections.[40]

15.1-20 Does the term *used* in <797> include the infusion time?

No. It means the time from compounding up to the point of initiation of administration.

15.1-21 How do I know to use the aseptic processing BUDs or the terminal sterilization BUDs?

The only way you can use the BUDs for terminal sterilization is if you use an autoclave, dry heat oven, or irradiation procedure. Mixing CSP components—even if you filter the CSP—is not terminal sterilization.

5.1-22 Is a summary of the maximum BUD times available?

See **Exhibits 15-1** through **15-6** based on the compounding facility and method used.

EXHIBIT 15-1. BUDs for Category 1 CSPs

BUD for Category 1 CSPs		
	Controlled Room Temperature	Refrigerated
Made from only sterile components	12 hours or less	24 hours or less
Made from one or more nonsterile component	12 hours or less	24 hours or less

BUD = beyond-use date, CSP = compounded sterile preparation.

EXHIBIT 15-2. BUDs for Aseptically Prepared Category 2 CSPs (Without a Sterility Test of the Final CSP) Made Only from Sterile Components

BUDs for Aseptically Prepared Category 2 CSPs Made only from Sterile Components No Sterility Test Performed or Passed			
	Controlled Room Temperature	Refrigerated	Frozen
BUD	4 days	10 days	45 days

BUD = beyond-use date, CSP = compounded sterile preparation.

EXHIBIT 15-3. BUDs for Aseptically Prepared Category 2 CSPs (Without a Sterility Test of the Final CSP) Made from One or More Nonsterile Component

BUDs for Aseptically Prepared Category 2 CSPs Made from One or More Nonsterile Components No Sterility Test Performed or Passed			
	Controlled Room Temperature	Refrigerated	Frozen
BUD	1 day	4 days	45 days

BUD = beyond-use date, CSP = compounded sterile preparation.

EXHIBIT 15-4. BUDs for Aseptically Prepared Category 2 CSPs That Have Passed the Requirements for Sterility Testing

BUDs for Aseptically Prepared Category 2 CSPs <797> Sterility Testing Passed			
	Controlled Room Temperature	Refrigerated	Frozen
BUD	30 days	45 days	60 days

BUD = beyond-use date, CSP = compounded sterile preparation.

EXHIBIT 15-5. BUDs for Terminally Sterilized Category 2 CSPs Without a Sterility Test Performed or Passed

BUDs for Terminally Sterilized Category 2 CSPs No Sterility Test Performed or Passed			
	Controlled Room Temperature	Refrigerated	Frozen
BUD	14 days	28 days	45 days

BUD = beyond-use date, CSP = compounded sterile preparation.

EXHIBIT 15-6. BUDs for Terminally Sterilized Category 2 CSPs That Have Passed Requirements for Sterility Testing

BUDs for Terminally Sterilized Category 2 CSPs <797> Sterility Testing Passed			
	Controlled Room Temperature	Refrigerated	Frozen
BUD	45 days	60 days	90 days

BUD = beyond-use date, CSP = compounded sterile preparation.

15.1-23 We reconstitute and freeze some antibiotic syringes. Can I keep them for 45 days, then move them to the refrigerator for another 10 days?

No. BUDs are not additive. In this situation, the frozen syringes need to be discarded 45 days after compounding if not used (or earlier if they are not stable for that long).

15.1-24 We reconstitute and refrigerate some antibiotic syringes and give them a 10-day BUD. If we take them out of the refrigerator on day 4, what is the room temperature BUD?

BUDs are not additive, so the maximum time you could use them for is 10 days refrigerated (if they are stable that long). In this situation, you could assign a room temperature stability of up to 4 days (if they are stable that long at room temperature). They would still be usable for 6 days refrigerated, but the maximum room temperature BUD is 4 days. However, many organizations use a more conservative approach and use a shorter BUD than permitted by <797>.

15.1-25 We warm some solutions (either before use or after compounding). What is the BUD for solutions placed in warmers?

You need to follow the manufacturer's information and place the solutions in a controlled temperature warmer. IV manufacturers have this information because surgical services often warm solutions.

15.1-26 Can I extend the BUDs beyond those listed in <797>?

Extending BUDs is only permitted if USP monographs are used. To use the BUD in the monograph, the CSP must be compounded as directed, using the same packaging, the same storage temperature and completion of any required testing.

15.1-27 I have published studies that have BUDs of 1 or 2 years. Can I use them?

You can use the studies for the preparation if appropriate, but you cannot extend the BUD beyond 90 days.

15.1-28 I have published studies that show 100% of the compound remaining on day 30. Can I extrapolate that information to use a longer BUD?

No, not without other information to support it. The authors may have stopped the study at day 30, so that's all they can report. Perhaps the compound is stable longer, but you have no proof of that.

15.1-29 Is it always OK to use the default dates listed in <797>?

No. Other factors may require you to use shorter times, including the following:

- How the CSP reacts over time
- The interaction of the container or closure with the CSP
- Microbial growth

15.1-30 If I make a CSP today, does the time for the BUD start today or tomorrow?

The BUD begins from the time the preparation is started.

15.1-31 Do BUDs for intrathecal or epidural CSPs need to be less than those defaults listed in <797>?

<797> does not distinguish among any specific sterile dosage form. However, many organizations use BUDs shorter than the allowable defaults, especially for dosage forms that are administered as intraspinal or ophthalmic drugs.

15.1-32 Pharmacy references often have stability information that is longer than the BUDs allowed in <797>. Can I use the references?

There are several valuable references often used, including ASHP's *Handbook of Injectable Drugs*,[41] Dellamorte Bing/Nowobilski-Vasilios's *Extended Stability for Parenteral Drugs*,[42] and King's *Guide to Parenteral Admixtures*.[43] These are references for stability. You need to use the *shorter* of stability (such as from the manufacturer, these references, or other peer-reviewed sources) or sterility limits as defined in <797> BUD tables.

15.1-33 My state has the old BUDs in regulations. Do I follow them or new <797> information?

Use the more conservative of the times.

15.1-34 Do the BUDs in <797> apply to compounds made for animals?

Yes. <797> applies to both human and animal nonsterile compounds. There is no distinction among species for BUD assignment.

15.1-35 Does the BUD differ based on the category of compound (low, medium, or high risk)?

Those categories were in a prior version of <797> and are not in the 2019 revision.

15.2 ACTIVE PHARMACEUTICAL INGREDIENTS AND OTHER COMPONENTS

15.2-1 What is the BUD of opened jars of components?

Active pharmaceutical ingredients (APIs) need to come from an FDA-registered supplier, so they will have an expiration date assigned by the manufacturer. For other components, mark the date when they are received, and assign a BUD no longer than 1 year from the date of receipt.

15.2-2 What should I do with old bottles of chemicals and other components?

Properly discard them.

15.2-3 Can the container used for the package of a CSP affect the stability?

Yes. Both the container and the closure used can affect stability.

15.3 VIAL/BAG SYSTEMS

15.3-1 What is the BUD of products like ADD-Vantage™, MiniBag Plus, VIAL-MATE, addEASE®, and similar systems?

If these are attached and activated for immediate use, it is considered preparation per approved labeling, not compounding. But in this case, you would be using it right away.

If the vials and bags are attached (docked), but not activated and will be stored for future use, it is considered compounding, so the personnel, facility, and other requirements of <797> must be met. Note that not all bag/vial systems are approved for docking, storage, and future use. For those that are approved for docking and future use, the BUD is not limited to the times in the default tables because manufacturers perform testing on these prior to Food and Drug Administration (FDA) approval. You can use the BUDs provided by the manufacturer that are based on the bag component remaining with the specifications for the fluid in the plastic container.

15.4 VIALS AND OTHER DOSAGE FORMS

15.4-1 Do BUDs apply to manufactured products, or only compounded preparations?

They apply to vials and other manufactured components if they are used on more than one occasion.

15.4-2 What is the BUD of a single-dose ampule?

A single-dose ampule must be discarded immediately after use.

15.4-3 What's the BUD of a single-dose vial?

If a single-dose vial is opened or punctured in ambient air, it must be discarded immediately after use. If a single-dose vial is opened or punctured in ISO 5 or cleaner air (such as inside a PEC), it may be used for up to 12 hours as long as the storage requirements from the manufacturer are followed.

15.4-4 Is a manufactured IV bag (like a saline bag used for reconstituting antibiotics) a single-dose or a multiple-dose container?

It is a single-dose container. If a parenteral container intended for single use is opened or punctured in ISO 5 or cleaner air (such as inside a primary engineering control [PEC]), it may be used for up to 12 hours as long as the storage requirements from the manufacturer are followed.

15.4-5 Once an IV is spiked, what is the BUD?

Once an IV is spiked, it should be used right away.

15.4-6 Is the BUD of a manufactured solution different from a compounded CSP?

Spiking and hanging a manufactured IV solution is not compounding, so <797> does not apply. You can use the manufacturer's expiration date, as long as the produce has been stored according to the manufacturer's instructions (e.g., proper temperature, intact packaging).

15.4-7 What's the BUD of an IV made during a code?

A CSP made at bedside during a code would be used right away. It needs to follow the immediate-use information in <797>.

15.4-8 When I go in the operating room (OR) prep room on evenings, I see several cases of IV solutions spiked and hanging. The OR says this is standard practice and there is no BUD. Is this correct?

This is not specifically addressed in <797> but is an issue of safe practice. Once an IV is spiked, it should be used right away. There are no preservatives in the solution. Your infection preventionist can help you eliminate this unsafe practice. Also see the Association for Professionals in Infection Control and Epidemiology (APIC) position paper on Safe Infection, Infusion, and Medication Vial Practices in Healthcare[25] for further information.

15.4-9 Is a manufactured irrigation bottle a single-dose or a multiple-dose container?

It is a single-dose container.

15.4-10 What is the BUD of a multiple-dose vial?

28 days unless otherwise specified in the product labeling.

15.4-11 Once punctured, should a multiple-dose vial be refrigerated or kept in the hood?

This is a stability, sterility, and patient safety issue. You need to follow the manufacturer's instructions for storage, including BUD and storage temperature. The Institute for

Safe Medication Practices (ISMP) has safety information about the risk of storing vials inside a PEC that are not being used for the preparation being mixed.[31] Establish your policy with all these issues in mind.

15.4-12 If I am going to save a multiple-dose vial for future use, do I need to date it with the open date or the end date?

You need to date it with the BUD. Your policy may specify additional requirements.

15.4-13 If a multiple-dose vial is missing the cap, does that affect the BUD?

Vial caps are dust covers for the stopper; they do not indicate a sterile septum. If you can be sure the vial has not been compromised, there is no difference if it has a cap or not. If this occurs more than rarely, it either needs to be reported to the FDA MedWatch program[44] if received from the supplier, or investigated thoroughly if it emanates from your storage area. It could be related to tampering of the drugs.

15.4-14 What is the BUD of a pharmacy bulk package (PBP)?

PBPs are single-dose vials containing many doses (e.g., a 10-g cefazolin vial or a 50-mL vial of an electrolyte intended for total parenteral nutrition [TPN] compounding). The PBP will have a BUD time in the product labeling that must be followed. PBPs may only be opened or punctured under ISO 5 or cleaner air (e.g., inside a PEC).

15.4-15 If a PBP is labeled with a manufacturer's in-use time of 4 hours, can I still use it for 12 hours since I opened it under the hood?

No. You need to follow the information in the product labeling.

15.5 COMPOUNDED STOCK BAGS

15.5-1 We mix an electrolyte bag to use in neonatal TPNs. How long is the bag good for?

There are a lot of different situations when stock bags are prepared, so be sure to refer to the full text in <797> for your specific situation. A common situation is preparing a stock bag in a cleanroom suite, adding one or more conventionally manufactured electrolytes into a manufactured IV solution. Once you mix the bag, you can store it (unused) for up to the allowed BUD based on the storage temperature. That could be as long as 10 days refrigerated if the mixture is stable that long. When you need to use it, puncture it inside the ISO 5 PEC and use it for up to 12 hours, then discard it.

The CSPs made from that stock bag could potentially have a BUD that is *no longer* than the BUD on the stock bag. For example, if your stock bag has a BUD of 10 days and you remove it from the refrigerator on day 5, the CSPs made with it could have a BUD of 5 days (if stable that long). If you remove the stock bag and puncture it on day 8, the CSPs made from it could have a BUD of 2 days (if stable that long). However, consider a more conservative approach, such as mixing smaller stock bags and using a shorter BUD. Many organizations mix a stock bag, use it that day (within 12 hours) and use a short BUD for the subsequently mixed CSPs, such as 24 hours.

15.5-2 Our 503B outsourcing facility mixes stock bags for us. Do they have a different BUD than if I mixed them myself?

Find out if your outsourcing facility has validated studies to support a BUD beyond which you would use. Make your decision on that, coupled with the requirements in <797>.

DISPENSING AND PACKAGING 16

(See Section 19 in USP <797>.)

16.1 What are some key issues to confirm when dispensing a compounded sterile preparation?

Check that the compounded sterile preparation (CSP) matches the order or prescription, the master formulation record (MFR), and the compounding record (CR), and check that it is labeled correctly. If the CSP was compounded in advance of dispensing, a visual check needs to be done to be sure it still meets the physician appearance expected. If the MFR requires specific testing (such as pH), be sure that is done and recorded.

16.2 What has to be on the label of a compounded sterile preparation?

The label on the immediate container needs to display at least the following:

- Assigned internal identification number (such as barcode, prescription or order number, or lot number)
- Active components, including amount/activity or concentration
- Dosage form
- Route of administration
- Amount or volume in the container if not obvious
- Storage temperature if other than controlled room temperature
- Beyond-use date
- Storage conditions if other than controlled room temperature
- If it is a single-dose container, a statement stating that when space permits
- If it is a multiple-dose container, a statement stating exactly that

The labeling on the CSP should include the following:

- Indication that the preparation is compounded
- Any special handling instructions
- Any applicable warning statements
- Name, address, and contact information of the compounding facility if the CSP will be sent outside the facility or healthcare system where it was compounded

Your state board or accreditation organization may have additional requirements.

16.3 What's the difference between the label and the labeling?

The *label* needs to be affixed to the final container. *Labeling* includes the label and any additional information except the outer shipping container.

16.4 Why would there be a different spot to put a label on a CSP?

The distinction between label and labeling is to allow for situations where the immediate container is too small for the entire labeling requirements. For example, you might make several 1-mL syringes or eye drops in small containers. Each dose needs to have the label requirements, but the rest of the information could be on a bag in which the syringes or eye drop bottles are placed.

16.5 Does a CSP label have to include the fact that it is compounded?

<797> says the labeling should include the fact that the preparation is compounded. Your state may have more stringent requirements.

16.6 Does the technician who mixed the CSP and the pharmacist who checked the CSP need to initial the label?

Define that in your policies and procedures. Ideally, an image of the label with that information (initialed either manually or electronically) would be available. But many organizations do not yet have the technology to support permanent electronic capture of that information. You need to have a method to identify the individuals involved in the compounding process and the person who verified the final CSP. That information needs to be retrievable after the CSP has been discarded.

16.7 Are there requirements for the packaging that must be used for CSPs that are mailed or shipped?

Your policies need to define how you will appropriately package CSPs that will be mailed or shipped. The packaging needs to be able to protect the integrity of the CSP and the safety of personnel who handle them.

16.8 Are temperature monitors required for CSPs that are shipped?

You need to determine that based on the CSP and shipping process.

CLEANING AND DISINFECTING 17

(See Section 7 in USP <797>.)

17.1 GENERAL INFORMATION

17.1-1 What is the difference between deactivating, decontaminating, cleaning, and disinfecting?

- *Deactivating* renders a substance inert.
- *Decontaminating* removes substances from the surface using a disposable wiper.
- *Cleaning* removes residue such as dirt from surfaces using a cleaning agent and manual process.
- *Disinfecting* is then done to ensure the surfaces are free from contamination.

17.1-2 <800> mentions decontaminating, but <797> doesn't. Why? Do I still need to decontaminate my chemo areas?

Yes. You need to decontaminate areas where hazardous drugs are handled. Decontamination isn't mentioned in <797> because all hazardous drug handling needs to comply with both <797> and <800>. See <800>[4] for those details.

17.1-3 <797> mentions use of sporicidals. Why?

These agents applied at an appropriate concentration for the contact (dwell) time listed in the product labeling destroy spores.

17.1-4 Which is done first: cleaning or disinfecting?

Cleaning is done first, then following by disinfecting surfaces. An Environmental Protection Agency (EPA)-registered one-step disinfectant cleaner may be able to be used according to the manufacturer's instructions to perform both steps in one application.

17.1-5 Do I need to wear garb when cleaning?

Yes. Cleaning inside the sterile compounding area requires the same garb as when compounding. In some cases, additional eye and respiratory protection may be needed. Many organizations include goggles to protect eyes when cleaning agents are used above waist level. Check the manufacturer's information for the solutions you are using for additional information specific to that chemical.

17.1-6 What does *dwell time* mean?

Dwell time is the amount of time a solution needs to be wet and in contact with the surface to meet the product claims. The dwell time for EPA-registered one-step disinfectant cleaning solutions is listed on the product labeling. Because of the air flow in the PECs and compounding suites, a long dwell time is impractical; the agent won't stay wet for the required time. A required dwell time more than 3 minutes may be impractical.

17.1-7 We always clean with sterile alcohol. Is that enough?

No. Alcohol is not a cleaner; it is a disinfectant/sanitizing agent. You need to use an agent that contains a detergent or surfactant to clean.

17.1-8 Is alcohol a sanitizing agent?

Yes. 70% sterile isopropyl alcohol (sIPA) is the sanitizing agent used when compounding sterile preparations.

17.1-9 Can an ultraviolet light be used to sanitize an area?

It cannot be used instead of 70% sterile isopropyl alcohol (sIPA).

7.1-10 Is sterile alcohol required in <797>?

Yes. When alcohol is used in or on the PEC or containers being placed in the PEC, 70% sterile isopropyl alcohol is required.

17.1-11 Should cleaning agents be rotated?

There is no requirement to rotate agents to combat the development of microbial resistance. Bactericidal cleaning agents are used as daily cleaners, but a sporicidal cleaning agent must be used monthly. This is not rotation per se, but a different agent is selected because it has different actions.

17.1-12 Are reusable mops acceptable to use?

They are not prohibited, but consider the process you use. Standardizing on disposable mop heads removes the concern of spreading contamination from one area to another.

17.1-13 What is the best way to monitor that cleaning has been done?

The designated person should monitor that this is done. Cleaning done daily or less frequently needs to be documented. Some state regulations require additional or more frequent documentation.

17.1-14 Do pharmacy personnel need to do all the cleaning of sterile compounding areas?

Only compounders with documented competence in sterile compounding can clean PECs and other sensitive equipment. Either pharmacy or environmental services staff can clean the rooms, but any personnel involved in cleaning sterile compounding areas needs to have documented competency. Regulators and accreditation organizations often expect pharmacy staff to oversee the training and confirm the competence of nonpharmacy personnel who clean sterile compounding areas.

17.1-15 When and with what do supplies going into the sterile compounding area need to be cleaned?

Your policies and procedures need to detail how the outside of containers (e.g., vials, boxes in which vials are packaged) are cleaned prior to placement in sterile compounding area. Drugs and supplies going into the buffer room or crossing over the perimeter line in an SCA must first be wiped with a sporicidal agent or a sterile disinfectant like sIPA. Immediately prior to placing drugs and other supplies in the PEC, the outside of each item must be wiped with sIPA. For supplies such as syringes that are received in sterile packaging, the outside of the package needs to be wiped; the sterile syringes inside the package do not if the package is opened as they are placed inside the PEC.

17.1-16 What is a one-step cleaner? Can I use these in the intravenous (IV) room?

Yes, you can. An EPA-registered one-step disinfectant cleaner means that both cleaning and disinfecting occur in one step. These solutions are not appropriate when dirty areas are cleaned, but that should not be an issue in a sterile compounding area other than cleaning on commissioning the area.

7.1-17 What cleaning and disinfecting needs to be done daily?

Daily cleaning and disinfecting needs to include the following:

- PEC
- Equipment inside PEC
- Surface of the removable work tray of the PEC
- Pass-throughs
- Work surfaces outside the PEC but inside the SEC
- Surfaces of sinks

Floors need to be cleaned daily but do not have to be disinfected with sIPA.

17.1-18 Does the PEC need to be cleaned and disinfected every 30 minutes?

The PEC surface needs to be sanitized (with sIPA) at least every 30 minutes if compounding takes less than 30 minutes. If compounding takes longer than 30 minutes, disinfect the work surface after compounding is completed.

17.1-19 What cleaning needs to be done weekly?

There is no specific weekly cleaning required in <797> but many organizations identify specific areas (for which <797> requires monthly cleaning) to be cleaned weekly. If you require that, be sure your procedures and logs accurately reflect that.

17.1-20 What cleaning needs to be done monthly?

Additional monthly cleaning and disinfecting must be performed with a sporicidal cleaning agent. Surfaces to be cleaned include the following:

- All interior surfaces of the PEC and equipment within the PEC (*note:* monthly cleaning and disinfecting inside the PEC is always at least two steps)
  - Application of an EPA-registered one-step sporicidal disinfectant cleaner, then
  - Wiping with sIPA after the cleaning agent dwell time has been achieved
- Cleaning, disinfecting, and application of a sporicidal underneath the removable work of the PEC
- Floors
- Sinks
- Walls
- Doors and door frames
- Ceiling in the compounding suite
  - <797> allows ceilings in segregated compounding areas to be cleaned, disinfected, and applied with a sporicidal when visibly soiled or when contamination is known or suspected. However, consider performing this monthly.
- Storage shelving, bins, and their contents
- Equipment used outside the PEC but within the SEC
- All surfaces of pass-throughs
- All surfaces of PECs and any furniture (e.g., tables, shelves, carts)

17.1-21 If my IV room isn't used every day, do I still need to clean it every day?

No. If compounding has not occurred in 24 hours, even if you left the room clean, the chapter requires you to perform daily cleaning before compounding is begun. If the sterile compounding area isn't used in a month, then perform the daily and monthly cleaning requirements prior to compounding. Your state board may have more stringent requirements.

17.1-22 Are there requirements for who can clean the IV room?

Yes. Only compounding personnel with documented competence in performing hand hygiene and garbing appropriate to the space as well as in performing cleaning activities can clean the PECs. Either pharmacy personnel or environmental services personnel can clean the SECs. Environmental services personnel do not need to perform gloved fingertip and thumb sampling, because they don't compound, but they do need to complete the other garbing and hand hygiene competencies. The designated person should oversee the competency requirements for any personnel outside the pharmacy as well as all compounding personnel.

17.1-23 How often does competency documentation for cleaning need to occur?

For personnel who clean but do not compound, initially and then minimally every 12 months. Compounding personnel need to document hand hygiene and garbing—including gloved fingertip and thumb tests—initially and every 6 months; that information would also demonstrate garbing competency for cleaning preparation. Competency for cleaning (knowledge of solutions and preparation, processes to use, etc.) must be consistent for both pharmacy and environmental personnel. Be sure to document any in-services throughout the year that deal with cleaning and, if personnel outside the pharmacy clean the SECs, be sure to include them in the in-servicing as well.

17.2 TYPES OF CLEANING SOLUTIONS

17.2-1 How do I know what cleaning solutions to select?

Sterile 70% isopropyl alcohol must be used to sanitize inside the PECs after cleaning has been performed. Select your decontamination and cleaning solutions by evaluating the availability (which may be related to your buying group options), safety (for both personnel and your surfaces), and effectiveness. Your infection control practitioner may be able to help with identifying appropriate solutions. Consider use of ready-to-use solutions rather than those you must dilute. The EPA-registered one-step disinfectant cleaners will have compatibility and contact time information.

17.2-2 How do I know I am using the correct dilutions of cleaning solutions?

Read the manufacturer's instructions. Ready-to-use solutions are the most convenient because they do not require dilution. Be sure that the solutions remain in contact with the surface for the appropriate contact (dwell) time. Only use agents where the manufacturers specify dwell time or contact time in their instructions for use.

17.2-3 Is sterile water a cleaning solution?

No. Water is not a cleaner, but it is used to dissolve residue in the PEC.

17.2-4 Is bleach a cleaning solution?

Not as a single agent. It is a sporicidal (when used in the appropriate concentration for the appropriate dwell time) but needs to be partnered with a surfactant or detergent to be considered a cleaner.

17.2-5 If bleach is used as a sporicidal agent, what strength should be used?

It needs to be at least 0.5%, which is often listed on products as 5,000 parts per million. The concentration can be found on the product labeling. However, because bleach is often diluted, be sure the final concentration doesn't fall below 0.5%.

17.2-6 Once bleach is diluted, how long is it good for?

It needs to be mixed daily.

17.2-7 Are ready-to-use solutions required?

They aren't required by <797>, but they are desirable. Ready-to-use products are already properly diluted, so provide a safe process for both patients (the concentration is correct) and personnel (because they don't have to mix potentially dangerous chemicals). If you use a concentrate mixed with water, this process must be documented each time a solution is mixed. Measuring devices must be provided and properly maintained. Sterile Water for Irrigation must be used if the resulting solution will be used inside of the PEC.

17.2-8 How should cleaning agents be applied?

It's best to apply the solutions to a disposable wiper or cleaning tool cover. Never spray into the HEPA filters and never in hazardous drug preparation as. In many cases, you will also need tools to reach the areas you need to clean. The reusable tool handles and holders need to be dedicated for use in the sterile compounding area; for hazardous drug rooms (buffer rooms and containment segregated compounding area [C-SCAs]), dedicate reusable tool handles and holders to only that area. The tool handles and holders need to be cleanable and cleaned and disinfected before and after each use. They cannot be made of wood or other particle-shedding material.

17.2-9 Can any type of cloth be used for the wiper?

No. Wipers need to be disposable and low-linting.

17.3 CLEANING PECs AND OTHER COMPOUNDING EQUIPMENT

17.3-1 How often should PECs and other equipment used for compounding be cleaned?

Any equipment used to compound should be cleaned as soon as possible once compounding is completed.

17.3-2 What types of solutions should be used for cleaning the hoods?

For PECs used for nonhazardous compounding, two steps are necessary:

1. Clean with a detergent, then
2. Wipe with sterile 70% IPA

For PECs used for hazardous drug compounding, three steps are necessary:

1. Decontaminate with an agent that has been verified to decontaminate HDs, then
2. Clean with a detergent, then
3. Wipe with sterile 70% IPA

You may need to use sterile water to remove visible particles prior to the cleaning step if debris or residue is present.

17.3-3 What does *terminal cleaning* mean?

It is not a term used in <797> nor an adequate description of the required process. (It comes from a patient care perspective; sterile compounding is a different process.) What it generally meant by this is the *monthly cleaning*, and that is the term that should be used.

17.3-4 Who should clean the hoods?

Only compounding personnel may decontaminate, clean, and disinfect the PECs and the equipment in them.

17.3-5 How often do the hoods or other compounding surfaces need to be cleaned during compounding?

Cleaning and sanitizing are different actions. First, the inside of PECs must be sanitized with sIPA at the beginning and end of each shift, after spills, and when surface contamination is known or suspected. The deck (flat surface) of the hood and work surfaces need to be sanitized between compounding CSPs with different components and more frequently if needed.

Cleaning and disinfection must be performed daily at the end of the compounding day (or at a defined time during the day if the sterile compounding area is used 24/7).

17.3-6 Do I have to clean the hoods even on days they are not used?

No. If the hood has not been used in more than 24 hours, then <797> says it must be cleaned and disinfected with a cleaning agent and then wiped with sterile IPA before use. If it was cleaned and less than 24 hours has elapsed, wipe all surfaces inside the hood with sIPA before use. Your policies and procedures need to reflect your actual process. If the hood is turned off or power is lost for any reason, then the daily cleaning and disinfection must be performed before it is used for sterile compounding.

17.3-7 How often does an automated compounding device need to be cleaned?

At least daily when it (or the PEC in which it resides) is cleaned. It may need to be cleaned more frequently if source containers spill on the components. Remember that this equipment is inside or close to the direct compounding area and must be wiped with sIPA as frequently as the PEC deck is wiped.

17.3-8 How often does a repeater pump need to be cleaned?

At least daily when it (or the PEC in which it resides) is cleaned. It may need to be cleaned more frequently if source containers spill on the components. Remember that this equipment is inside or close to the direct compounding area and must be wiped with sIPA as frequently as the PEC deck is wiped.

17.3-9 How often does any computer equipment need to be cleaned?

At least daily when it (or the PEC in which it resides) is cleaned. It may need to be cleaned more frequently if there are spills or drips on the components. Remember that this equipment is inside or close to the direct compounding area and must be wiped with sIPA as frequently as the PEC deck is wiped.

17.3-10 If the power goes off, do we need to clean the hoods?

Yes. Anytime power is lost to a PEC or is turned off all interior surfaces of the PEC and anything residing on the PEC deck must be cleaned and disinfected with an EPA-registered one-step sporicidal cleaner and then those surfaces wiped with sIPA after the dwell time of the sporicidal has been achieved. Define that in your policies and procedures.

17.3-11 Do we need to clean syringes as we take them out of the packages?

No. Sterile supplies in sterile packaging do not need to be cleaned as long as the outside of the packages are clean, and they are opened inside the PEC.

17.4 CLEANING COMPOUNDING AREAS

17.4-1 Is it OK for environmental services personnel to clean the floors while we are compounding?

No. Cleaning cannot occur while you are compounding.

17.4-2 Is alcohol sufficient to clean the compounding areas?

No. Alcohol is neither a decontaminating agent nor a cleaner. Alcohol is a disinfectant when the required dwell time is reached and is useful only after cleaning has occurred inside PECs.

17.4-3 Who should clean the compounding area?

Either compounding personnel or environmental services personnel can clean the compounding area floors, walls, and ceilings. Training and documented competence is required. In any case, all compounding personnel should be competent in this task in case environmental services personnel are not available. Regulatory agencies and accreditation organizations often expect pharmacy to oversee the competency of nonpharmacy employees who clean the compounding area.

17.4-4 What is a "high-touch" area?

Areas that are frequently touched, like carts, counters, refrigerators, pass-throughs, door handles, etc.

17.4-5 Do I have to clean the compounding area even on days it is not used?

No, but be sure to clean the hood and compounding areas before you begin compounding. Your policies and procedures need to reflect your actual process.

17.4-6 How often does the office space inside the anteroom need to be cleaned?

If you mean a counter where staging of supplies occurs, that needs to be cleaned at least daily. If you mean space for administrative activities, that should not be occurring in the anteroom or buffer room. If you perform activities that could be done outside the sterile compounding area, take steps to improve that process and in the meantime, clean more frequently than required.

17.4-7 How often do pass-throughs need to be cleaned?

Daily.

17.4-8 How often do refrigerators in the sterile compounding area need to be cleaned?

As often as necessary to keep them clean. Also perform viable air sampling near them in to ensure they are not compromising your microbial state of control.

17.4-9 Because I compound only occasionally, do I have to clean my whole pharmacy with the same frequency as the compounding area?

<797> deals only with sterile compounding. Your state board regulations may have additional information.

17.4-10 How often should I use alcohol to clean the floor?

Alcohol is *not* a cleaner; it is a sanitizing/disinfecting agent. There is no value in using alcohol or sterile alcohol for this purpose. Use a detergent to clean the floor.

17.5 CLEANING SUPPLIES NEEDED FOR COMPOUNDING

17.5-1 When and with what should drug vials, IV bags, needles, and syringes be cleaned?

This is a process involving several steps. If a hazardous drug is received (all NIOSH Table 1 antineoplastics[18] and any other National Institute for Occupational Safety and Health (NIOSH) hazardous drugs that have not been entity-exempt in the organization's Assessment of Risk need to be wiped prior to the location where they will be stored. For Table 1 hazardous drugs, you should be receiving the drugs enclosed in impervious plastic within the tote or other shipping container. See <800>[4] and *The Chapter <800> Answer Book*[8] for information.

For nonhazardous drugs and supplies, use the following steps:

1. Prior to taking drugs, IVs, and other supplies into the clean side of the anteroom, into pass-throughs, or inside the perimeter of the SCA or C-SCA, wipe the outside of the package with a sporicidal agent, EPA-registered disinfectant, or sIPA. Be sure that the process you use does not obliterate any labeling on the product, such as lot number and expiration date.

2. Right before the drugs, IVs, or supplies are placed in the PEC, wipe the outside of the vial, IV bag or overwrap, outside of the packaging of sterile supplies, or other component with sIPA. Allow the sIPA to dry. Do not wipe the syringes, needles, IV sets, and other sterile components that come packaged as sterile items as long as the package is opened inside the PEC.

3. Critical sites (vial stoppers, necks of ampules, IV bag ports, etc.) exposed in the PEC must be wiped with sIPA before puncturing or entering the component.

ENVIRONMENTAL MONITORING 18

(See Section 6 in USP <797>.)

18.1 GENERAL INFORMATION

18.1-1 What is environmental monitoring?

The process by which facilities are evaluated and tested to ensure maintenance of a state of control. In <797>, it concerns viable monitoring.

18.1-2 Is environmental monitoring the same as certification?

No. They are different. Certification is the process of validating the nonviable elements of your PEC and SEC, including particle counts, air flow and pattern evaluation, pressure gradients, and other parameters that a compounding area is expected to maintain. *Environmental monitoring* is the testing and evaluation of viable (bacterial and fungal) sources of potential contamination.

18.1-3 Our environmental monitoring is done by our certifier. Is that OK?

You, your certifier, or other qualified personnel can perform the monitoring.

18.1-4 Does our environmental monitoring have to be done by our certifier?

No. It can be done by you, your certifier, or other qualified personnel.

18.1-5 What does viable monitoring do?

It detects microbial contamination.

18.1-6 I thought only the certifier could do air sampling. Is that correct?

No. It can be done by you, your certifier, or other qualified personnel. An independent certifier needs to certify your primary engineering controls (PECs) and secondary engineering controls (SECs), and that includes air sampling for particles. The air and surface sampling done for viable environmental monitoring is different.

18.1-7 Do I need a detailed policy, or can I depend on what my certifier does?

Certification checks nonviable elements; environmental monitoring is different. Your certifier may perform environmental monitoring for you, but you need to provide the certifier with your policies and monitoring plan.

18.1-8 Do hoods and rooms need to be tested before they are used?

Yes, tested and acceptable results returned. You need to be sure your PECs and SECs are in a state of control prior to using them for sterile compounding.

18.1-9 How often does environmental monitoring need to be done?

Electronic air sampling by impaction and surface sampling must be done initially to establish baseline levels of quality and to be sure the area is in a state of control. Following the commissioning of your sterile compounding area, electronic air sampling must be done at least every 6 months and surface sampling must be done at least monthly. That needs to be supplemented by follow-up monitoring if your areas show growth above the action level or when you want to trend the results for more robust monitoring.

18.1-10 What does *commissioning* mean?

Commissioning means checking your sterile compounding area prior to compounding in that area to be sure the space is in a state of control: the PECs and SECs are operating correctly, all equipment has undergone checks required by the manufacturer's specifications, there is no concerning microbial contamination in the area, etc.

18.1-11 What is a sampling plan?

The sampling plan is your policy and procedure that details what samples will be taken, what media will be used, how the samples will be incubated, how the incubator temperature is controlled and monitoring, how action levels will be addressed, and other details that will allow you to assess the state of control of the sterile compounding area.

18.1-12 What is an action level?

An action level is the level above which you need to take action. The action taken is intended to correct the reason you had microbial growth.

18.1-13 What is an alert level?

Alert levels aren't defined in <797>, but you may want to set an alert level, which needs to be lower than the action level, to indicate a trigger for specific requirements in your monitoring policy.

18.1-14 What are highly pathogenic organisms?

Highly pathogenic organisms are any organism that could be an issue to a susceptible patient. That term was used in the previous version of <797> but is not used in the 2019 version.

18.1-15 What is a CFU?

A CFU is a colony-forming unit. Each distinct colony on a media plate is 1 CFU.

18.1-16 Do I have to test for fungus if I don't make any high-risk preparations?

The risk levels are no longer part of <797>. All sterile compounding PECs and SECs must be tested for both bacterial and fungal contamination.

18.1-17 Do I have to incubate the samples?

Yes. The samples need to be incubated at a controlled temperature in an incubator.

18.1-18 Do I need an incubator in the pharmacy?

You need to be sure the samples are appropriately incubated. That might be done in your department (although do not place the incubator in the sterile compounding area), by your laboratory, or by an outside laboratory (which may be contracted by you or your certifier).

18.1-19 Is a warmer OK to use to incubate the samples?

No. You need to use an incubator.

18.1-20 Can I use the mannitol warmer to incubate the samples?

No. You need to use an incubator to incubate the samples at the temperature required in <797>. You certainly don't want to mix drugs with samples of growth media in the same device.

18.1-21 Does the incubator need special controls?

The device needs to be intended for use in incubating growth media. The temperature must be maintained and documented via continuous recording (preferred) or manually. The incubator must be outside the sterile compounding area and should be attached to emergency power.

18.1-22 Can the microbiology laboratory at the hospital incubate the samples?

They may be able to incubate the surface samples but probably not the air samples. Hospital laboratories are set up to handle patient samples, not environmental samples. Keep in mind that many have limited resources, so may not be able to take on the additional burden and may not have incubator space. If incubator space is the only issue, consider purchasing the incubator for the microbiology department to use for pharmacy samples.

18.1-23 Can an outside laboratory incubate the samples?

Yes, and this is often done by certifiers. The laboratory should be accredited to ISO 17025, which is the standard used by testing and calibration laboratories. The chain of custody of the samples is important to maintain.

18.1-24 Who should identify the growth?

A qualified individual such as a microbiologist.

18.1-25 Can I incubate the samples in the pharmacy and send them to the laboratory for identification?

Discuss this with your microbiology department. In some organizations, the incubator for the samples is stored in the pharmacy department but not in the sterile compounding area. If growth is found, a microbiologist could identify the organisms. The chain of custody for the samples is important to maintain.

18.1-26 Can I incubate the samples in the pharmacy and identify them myself?

The identification of microorganisms needs to be done with the assistance of a microbiologist. See *USP General Chapter <1113> Microbial Characterization, Identification, and Strain Typing.*[45] The chain of custody for the samples is important to maintain.

18.1-27 Does it really matter what is growing or is just the fact that there are a lot of CFUs on the plate enough information?

If the action level is exceeded, you need to attempt to identify the microorganism to the genus level with the assistance of a microbiologist.

18.1-28 What does *TNTC* mean on my microbiology report?

TNTC means too numerous to count. A report of TNTC is clearly above the action level.

18.2. ACTIVE AIR SAMPLING

18.2-1 What does *active air sampling* mean?

Use of an electronic sampling method that is done by impaction. A measured volume of air is drawn into a device that contains an agar plate. Any microbial contamination will be captured on the plate, which is then incubated.

18.2-2 What device is used to sample the air?

A microbial air sampler is the device used.

18.2-3 What is measured by active air sampling?

Microbial contamination in the PEC and SEC.

18.2-4 What has to be sampled?

Any ISO-classified space: all PECs, compounding suites (both anterooms and buffer rooms), and any high efficiency particulate air (HEPA)-filtered pass-through chamber.

18.2-5 How often is active air sampling required?

Initially to established baseline levels of quality and to be sure the area is in a state of control. Then, the minimum frequency is every 6 months. (If your certifier does this for you, it will likely be done at the same time as the certification of the PECs and SECs.) If growth above the action level is found, you will need to sample after remediation to be sure whatever caused the excursion has been corrected.

18.2-6 Do settling plates comply with <797>?

No. Settling plates are a passive test. You need to use active air sampling to comply with <797>.

18.2-7 Do I have to sample the air in pass-throughs?

If it is a HEPA-filtered pass-through, it needs to be sampled because it is an ISO classified area.

18.2-8 What media is used?

<797> allows two approaches. Trypticase soy agar (TSA) can be used for both bacterial and fungal sampling, or one sample can be TSA and the other a suitable fungal media, such as malt extract agar (MEA) or Sabouraud dextrose agar (SDA).

18.2-9 What is the temperature required for incubators?

Two temperature ranges are required in <797>: 30–35°C, then 20–25°C. Some organizations use one incubator and adjust the temperature as described in <797>, and some organizations have two incubators, one set at each temperature range.

18.2-10 For how long are the samples incubated?

It depends on the process used. If one sample is incubated at two different temperatures, at least 7 days is required. See <797> Box 6-1 for details.[3]

18.2-11 What are the action levels for active air sampling?

The levels are different for each ISO classified area. See **Exhibit 18-1**.

EXHIBIT 18-1. Action Levels for Microbial Air Sampling

ISO Class	Action Level per Plate
5	More than 1 CFU per cubic meter of air
7	More than 10 CFU per cubic meter of air
8	More than 100 CFU per cubic meter of air

CFU = colony-forming unit.

18.3 SURFACE SAMPLING

18.3-1 What does *surface sampling* mean?

Surface sampling means sampling the surfaces exposed to sterile compounding with a plate containing growth media. Any microbial contamination will be captured on the plate, which is then incubated.

18.3-2 What device is used for surface sampling?

For flat surfaces, use a contact plate. It has a convex surface that extends above the lip of the plate. For surfaces that are not flat (such as junctures of surfaces, equipment, etc.), a swab can be used.

18.3-3 What is measured by surface sampling?

Microbial contamination on the surfaces.

18.3-4 How often is surface sampling required?

Initially to established baseline levels of quality and to be sure the area is in a state of control. Then, the minimum frequency is monthly. However, if growth above the action level is found, you will need to sample after remediation to be sure whatever caused the excursion has been corrected.

18.3-5 What surfaces have to be sampled?

All ISO-classified surfaces and pass-through chambers. The PEC deck (surface), the equipment in a PEC (such as a repeater pump, automated compounding device, workflow hardware, etc.), staging areas near the PEC (such as carts or counters), and frequently touched surfaces (such as counters, carts, pass-throughs, refrigerator handles, etc.) need to be included in the plan.

18.3-6 Do areas in the segregated compounding area (SCA) or containment segregated compounding area (C-SCA) have to be tested?

The PEC does. Consider testing areas within the perimeter of the PEC to be sure you are not compromising patient safety with contamination. However, testing the areas in the SCA or the C-SCA outside the PEC is not required by <797>. Note that you are likely to see growth, because the SCA or C-SCA does not have the controls of a cleanroom suite (such as ISO classification and HEPA-filtered ceiling air). Action levels are not applied to the samples collected in the SCA or C-SCA.

18.3-7 When is the sampling done?

At least monthly at the end of compounding activities or end of shift but before the area has been cleaned and disinfected.

18.3-8 What areas are most likely to be at risk of contamination?

Surfaces where supplies are placed and other spots where activity occurs in the sterile compounding area.

18.3-9 What media is used?

A general microbial growth media (such as TSA) that has been supplemented with a neutralizer such as lecithin and polysorbate 80.

18.3-10 Our laboratory doesn't stock the media listed in <797>. Can regular or blood agar plates be used?

No. You need to use a media that includes neutralizers so you won't get false negative results from residual disinfecting agents. Laboratory suppliers can provide the media you need.

18.3-11 What is the temperature required for incubators?

Two temperature ranges are required in <797>: 30–35°C, then 20–25°C. Some organizations use one incubator and adjust the temperature as described in <797>, and some organizations have two incubators, one set at each temperature range.

18.3-12 For how long are the samples incubated?

It depends on the process used. If one sample is incubated at two different temperatures, at least 7 days is required. See <797> Box 6-2 for details.[3]

18.3-13 Are plates required for surface sampling or are paddles OK?

Plates, paddles, or slides can be used. Plates are appropriate for flat surfaces. Swabs are appropriate for other surfaces; the sampling swab may need to be plated. Check the manufacturer's information and the details in <797>.

18.3-14 Is there a special type of plate to use for surface sampling?

Yes. Contact plates (i.e., RODAC™ [Replicate Organism Detection and Counting] plates are used. They have a convex (not flat) surface.

18.3-15 Should I sample the same places each month or rotate areas?

Create a map of your sterile compounding area and mark the areas to test. You need to collect enough data to trend. Trended data should be evaluated at least annually and at that time, modifying sample locations may be appropriate based on the data.

18.3-16 What are the action levels for surface sampling?

The levels are different for each ISO classified area. See **Exhibit 18-2.**

EXHIBIT 18-2. Action Levels for Surface Sampling

ISO Class	Action Level per Plate or Swab
5	More than 3 CFU
7	More than 5 CFU
8	More than 50 CFU

CFU = colony-forming unit.

18.4 REACTING TO OUT-OF-SPECIFICATION RESULTS

18.4-1 What do I do when results are above the action level?

Action level excursions require you to look at the possible causes and attempt to remediate them.

18.4-2 Do I need to retest when out of specification results are found?

Yes. Once you have taken steps to remediate the issue, you need to retest to be sure the situation has been corrected.

18.4-3 There is 1 CFU of mold in the anteroom. What should I do?

Anterooms are the transition spaces between unclassified (not ISO classified) and controlled areas. It is not unusual to have some growth in the anteroom, even from mold. Even if the result is under the action level, you need to know that you have taken all appropriate steps to remediate what you can.

Some things to consider:
- Look at the location where the mold was found. Is it in the air or in a surface sample?
- Is this a repeated issue? If so, was the prior location the same?
- Is it near the sink?
- Is it near the entrance?
- Is it in or near a pass-through?
- Is it close to the refrigerator?

Determining sources can help you identify an appropriate remediation.

18.4-4 Where are likely sources of contamination?

Personnel, touch contamination, supplies, poor technique, work surfaces, and the air handling system are potential sources of contamination.

18.4-5 There is mold in the buffer room, but it's below the action level. What should I do?

Is this the first time you've found this, or is it a frequent occurrence? It is 1 CFU or always close to the action level? You need to evaluate the significance and frequency. Certainly, one immediate action is to check your cleaning practices and solutions. Be sure that you are using a sporicidal. Consider increasing the frequency of use of the sporicidal. (<797> requires this monthly but consider use weekly.) If it is a negative pressure buffer room, be sure that the pressure is within the range of negative 0.010 to 0.030″ to adjacent space. A room that is too negative can pull in contamination from adjacent space (including the ceiling). Check your most recent certification report to be sure the integrity of the HEPA filters were recorded, and don't indicate a potential problem. Involve your infection control practitioner in the evaluation. Perhaps he or she has found similar contamination in other areas in your organization.

18.4-6 My hood is OK, but my room isn't. What can I do until the room passes?

Unless there is an egregious situation in your SEC that you want to avoid using it or the PEC in it at all, you can consider this situation an SCA. You are then limited to Category 1 CSPs, including the limited BUD of 12 hours room temperature or 24 hours refrigerated. Your state board of pharmacy may have additional requirements.

18.4-7 What results do we have to report to our state board of pharmacy?

That depends on your state regulations. Be sure you are aware if and when you need to report excursions to the state board, other regulatory agency, or to a process defined in your policies and procedures.

QUALITY ASSURANCE AND QUALITY CONTROL 19

(See Section 18 in USP <797>.)

19.1 What is the difference between quality control and quality assurance?

Quality control are the processes you check following compounding to be sure the compounded sterile preparation (CSP) is within the specifications you intend. It might include pH, color, specific testing, or other checks. *Quality assurance* is a system of processes developed so you can be sure the compounds meet the appropriate quality standards.

19.2 Does <797> define the characteristics I need to follow?

See *USP General Chapter <1163> Quality Assurance in Pharmaceutical Compounding*[46] for information on the elements you should include in your policies.

19.3 Are the components of a QA program limited to the CSPs?

They are related to the compounds but encompass more than that. For example, you need to be able to identify patient complaints, adverse drug reactions, and medication errors related to the CSPs. The designated person needs to oversee the system to be sure it complies with your policies and procedures, could detect problems, and appropriately addresses issues.

19.4 What kinds of elements should we include on the report we present at the Infection Control Committee meeting?

This depends on the scope of your committee. Summary information should be reported to the appropriate committee (e.g., Infection Control, Quality, Pharmacy and Therapeutics). Be sure to report at the frequency defined in policy. Include those intervals when all results were within range considered acceptable (not just when issues are found).

Consider the following items in your report:

- Certification results, such as the status of the PECs and SECs (i.e., passed, failed, needs attention)
- Summary results of daily facility monitoring (e.g., number of days with acceptable readings, action taken for out of specification results)
- Number of personnel oriented to sterile compounding
- Personnel testing results (e.g., 9 out of 10 tests were within acceptable limits; 1 person was retested and waiting for results)

- Results of environmental monitoring (e.g., number of samples taken and percentage of results within acceptable limits, action taken on samples above the action level)

19.5 What are considered insanitary conditions?

The Food and Drug Administration (FDA) document *Insanitary Conditions at Compounding Facilities*[47] details the type of excursions considered unsanitary.

They include the following:

- Insects or rodents observed in or near compounding areas
- Visible contamination (both microbial and nonmicrobial)
- Handling different types of drugs without adequate separation to avoid cross-contamination
- Poor aseptic practices
- Storing open sterile containers without protective covers
- Use of nonsterile or nondepyrogenated containers or closures for sterile compounding
- Improper design or maintenance of the sterile compounding facility
- Insufficient sterilization time
- Use of improper filters
- Poor cleaning processes

Be sure your QA program addresses all of these issues.

WHAT DO I DO NOW?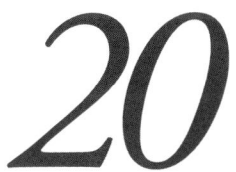

20.1 I'm overwhelmed with this information. Where do I start?

- Read <797>. There are also sterile compounding components in <800> and <825>.
- Perform a gap analysis. Compare the requirements (*must* statements) and recommendations (*should* statements) in <797> with your current practices.
- Assign a designated person and provide needed resources (e.g., educational programs).
- Examine your certification report, discuss noncompliant issues with your certifier, and take steps to become compliant. Identify the facility issues you need to improve and obtain administrative approval for any renovations needed.
- Work with your designated person to ensure personnel training and policy development.
- Ensure your policies and procedures are appropriate.
- Be sure key individuals at your organization—the person to whom you report, the risk manager, others as appropriate—are aware of noncompliant issues for which you need resources.

20.2 Is there a template action plan I could use to start assessing the compliance at my organization?

Exhibit 20-1 is an example of an action plan.

EXHIBIT 20-1. Example Action Plan for Compliance with USP <797>

	Element	Assigned To	Completed
List of CSPs			
Designated person			
Personnel training			
Garb	Gloves		
	Gowns		
	Other components		
Receiving	Training		
	Assess integrity of packages		
	Spill kit		
Sterile components and supply storage area			
Sterile compounding area			
Cleaning			
Quality assurance plan			

CSPs = compounded sterile preparations.

FUTURE EDITIONS

Do you have questions that were not answered? Feel free to submit questions that can be included in the next edition of this publication. Send the questions to publications@ashp.org.

REFERENCES

1. United States Pharmacopeial Convention (USP). *Compounding Compendium.* Rockville, MD: USP; 2019.
2. United States Pharmacopeial Convention (USP). USP general chapter <795> pharmaceutical compounding—nonsterile preparations. In: *USP 42–NF 37.* Second supplement. Rockville, MD: USP; 2019.
3. United States Pharmacopeial Convention (USP). USP general chapter <797> pharmaceutical compounding—sterile preparations. In: *USP 42–NF 37.* Second supplement. Rockville, MD: USP; 2019.
4. United States Pharmacopeial Convention (USP). USP general chapter <800> hazardous drugs—handling in healthcare settings. In: *USP 42–NF 37.* Second supplement. Rockville, MD: USP; 2019.
5. United States Pharmacopeial Convention (USP). USP general chapter <825> radiopharmaceuticals—preparation, compounding, dispensing, and repackaging. In: *USP 42–NF 37.* Second supplement. Rockville, MD: USP; 2019.
6. Newton DW. United States Pharmacopeia chapter <797> timeline 1989 to 2013. *Int J Pharm Compd.* 2013; 17:283-8.
7. US Food and Drug Administration. Repackaging of certain human drug products by pharmacies and outsourcing facilities, 2017. www.fda.gov/downloads/Drugs/Guidances/UCM434174.pdf (accessed 2019 Oct 17).
8. Kienle PC. *The chapter <800> answer book.* 2nd ed. Bethesda, MD: ASHP, 2020.
9. United States Pharmacopeial Convention (USP). USP general chapter <1168> compounding for phase 1 investigational studies. In: *USP 42–NF 37.* Second supplement. Rockville, MD: USP; 2019.
10. US Food and Drug Administration. Compounded drug products that are essentially copies of a commercially available drug product under section 503a of the Federal Food, Drug, and Cosmetic Act, 2018. www.fda.gov/downloads/Drugs/GuidanceComplianceRegulatoryInformation/Guidances/UCM510154.pdf (accessed 2019 Oct 17).
11. American Society of Health-System Pharmacists. ASHP sterile products preparation certificate program, 2019. www.ashp.org (accessed 2019 Oct 17).
12. CriticalPoint, LLC. Website. www.criticalpoint.info (accessed 2019 Oct 17).
13. Board of Pharmacy Specialties. BPS board certified sterile compounding pharmacist (BCSCP). www.bpsweb.org (accessed 2019 Oct 17).
14. Pharmacy Technician Certification Board. Certified compounded sterile preparation technician™ program. www.ptcb.org/about-ptcb/news-room/whats-new-at-ptcb/2017/12/06/ptcb-launches-certified-compounded-sterile-preparation-technician-(cspt)-program (accessed 2019 Oct 17).
15. Murdaugh LB. *Competence assessment tools for health-system pharmacies.* 5th ed. Bethesda, MD: American Society of Health-System Pharmacists; 2015.
16. American Society of Health-System Pharmacists (ASHP). ASHP's pharmacy competency assessment center. Bethesda, MD: ASHP; 2019.
17. United States Department of Labor, Occupational Safety and Health Administration. Hazard communication. www.osha.gov/dsg/hazcom/HCSFinalRegTxt.html (accessed 2019 Oct 17).
18. Centers for Disease and Control Prevention. NIOSH list of antineoplastic and other hazardous drugs in healthcare settings, 2016. Publication number 2016-161. www.cdc.gov/niosh/docs/2016-161/pdfs/2016-161.pdf (accessed 2019 Oct 17).
19. United States Department of Labor, Occupational Safety and Health Administration. Hazard communication: small entity compliance guide for employers that use hazardous chemicals. www.osha.gov/Publications/OSHA3695.pdf (accessed 2019 Oct 17).
20. Centers for Disease Control and Prevention. Hand hygiene in healthcare settings. www.cdc.gov/handhygiene (accessed 2019 Oct 17).
21. ASTM International. ASTM D6978 standard practice for assessment of resistance of medical gloves to permeation by chemotherapy drugs. www.astm.org/Standards/D6978.htm (accessed 2019 Oct 17).

22. ASTM International. ASTM F739 standard test for permeation of liquids and gases through protective clothing materials under conditions of continuous contact. www.astm.org/Standards/F739.htm (accessed 2019 Oct 17).

23. Centers for Disease Control and Prevention, National Institute for Occupational Safety and Health. The national personal protective technology laboratory, respirator trusted-source information. www.cdc.gov/niosh/npptl/topics/respirators/disp_part/respsource.html (accessed 2019 Oct 17).

24. Centers for Disease Control and Prevention. Safe injection practices to prevent transmission of infections to patients. www.cdc.gov/injectionsafety/ip07_standardprecaution.html (accessed 2019 Oct 17).

25. Association of Professionals in Infection Control and Epidemiology. APIC position paper: safe injection, infusion, and medication vial practices in health care (2016). www.apic.org/Resource_/TinyMceFileManager/Position_Statements/2016APICSIPPositionPaper.pdf (accessed 2019 Oct 17).

26. Buchanan C, Schneider P, Forrey R. *Compounding sterile preparations*. 4th ed. Bethesda, MD: American Society of Health-System Pharmacists; 2017.

27. United States Pharmacopeial Convention (USP) general chapter <71> sterility tests. In: *USP 42–NF 37*. Second supplement. Rockville, MD: USP; 2019.

28. US Food and Drug Administration. FD&C Act provisions that apply to human drug compounding. www.fda.gov/Drugs/GuidanceComplianceRegulatoryInformation/PharmacyCompounding/ucm606955.htm (accessed 2019 May 20).

29. United States Pharmacopeial Convention (USP). USP general chapter <1231> water for pharmaceutical purposes. In: *USP 42-NF 37*. Second supplement. Rockville, MD: USP; 2019.

30. Controlled Environment Testing Association. CETA application guides. www.cetainternational.org (accessed 2019 Oct 19).

31. Institute for Safe Medication Practices. Guidelines for safe preparation of compounded sterile preparations. www.ismp.org/guidelines/sterile-compounding (accessed 2019 Oct 17).

32. United States Pharmacopeial Convention (USP). USP general chapter <659> packaging and storage requirements. In: *USP 42–NF 37*. Second supplement. Rockville, MD: USP; 2019.

33. US Food and Drug Administration. Bulk drug substances used in compounding under section 503a of the FD&C Act. www.fda.gov/Drugs/GuidanceComplianceRegulatoryInformation/PharmacyCompounding/ucm614204.htm (accessed 2019 Oct 17).

34. US Food and Drug Administration. Regulatory policy information. www.fda.gov/drugs/human-drug-compounding/regulatory-policy-information (accessed 2019 Oct 17).

35. United States Pharmacopeial Convention (USP). USP general chapter <1178> good repackaging practices. In: *USP 42–NF 37*. Second supplement. Rockville, MD: USP; 2019.

36. American Society of Health-System Pharmacists. ASHP guidelines on compounding sterile preparations. *Am J Health-Syst Pharm*. 2014; 71:145-66.

37. Power LA, Coyne JW. ASHP guidelines on handling hazardous drugs. *Am J Health-Syst Pharm*. 2018; 75:1996-2031.

38. Centers for Disease Control and Prevention. Biosafety in microbiological and biomedical laboratories (BMBL). 5th ed. www.cdc.gov/labs/BMBL.html (accessed 2019 Oct 17).

39. International Journal of Pharmaceutical Compounding. Website. www.ijpc.com (accessed 2019 Oct 17).

40. Centers for Disease Control and Prevention. Guidelines for the prevention of intravascular catheter-related infections. www.cdc.gov/mmwr/preview/mmwrhtml/mm5132a9.htm (accessed 2019 Oct 17).

41. American Society of Health-System Pharmacists (ASHP). *Handbook on injectable drugs*. 20th ed. Bethesda, MD: ASHP; 2018.

42. Dellamorte Bing C, Nowobilski-Vasilios A. *Extended stability for parenteral drugs*. 6th ed. Bethesda, MD: American Society of Health-System Pharmacists; 2017.

43. King Guide Publications, Inc. *King guide to parenteral admixtures*. Napa, CA: King Guide Publications; 2019.

44. US Food and Drug Administration. MedWatch: the FDA safety information and adverse event reporting program. www.fda.gov/safety/medwatch-fda-safety-information-and-adverse-event-reporting-program (accessed 2019 Oct 17).

45. United States Pharmacopeial Convention (USP). USP general chapter <1113> microbial characterization, identification, and strain typing. In: *USP 42-NF 37*. Second supplement. Rockville, MD: USP; 2019.

46. United States Pharmacopeial Convention (USP). USP general chapter <1163> quality assurance in pharmaceutical compounding. In: *USP 42-NF 37*. Second supplement. Rockville, MD: USP; 2019.

47. US Food and Drug Administration. Insanitary conditions at compounding facilities. www.fda.gov/media/124948/download (accessed 2019 Oct 17).

INDEX

A

action level, 7, 44–45, 48, 124, 127–128, 130–131
action plan, 135–136
active air sampling, 123, 126–128
active pharmaceutical ingredients (APIs), 23, 51–52, 89
    beyond-use dates (BUDs) of, 106–107
addEASE®, 89, 107
ADD-Vantage™, 89, 107
administration, medication, 11
    defined, 33
    immediate use and preparation for, 33–36
air changes per hour (ACPH), 58, 59, 62, 64, 69
air flow, 37, 58
air handling system capacity, 62
albumin, 91
alcohol as disinfectant/sanitizing agent, 114, 120
alcohol-based hand gel, 24
alert level, 124
allergenic extracts, 7, 36, 95
allergenic extracts compounding area (AECA), 76–77
allergens, 4, 7
amber dropper bottles, 91
American Chemical Society (ACS) marking, 52
anesthesia personnel, 36
animals, application of USP <797> to, 9
anterooms, 64–67, 68, 79
    mold in, 131
    office space cleaning, 121
    pass-through chambers to, 72
    pressure in, 81
antibiotic CSPs, 92, 105
antibiotic vials, reconstitution of, 34
Appendix, USP <797>, 7
Aseptic Compounding Technique: Learning and Mastering the Ritual, 39
aseptic technique, 37
    beyond-use dates (BUDs) and, 102
    training in, 45–46
ASHP Guidelines on Compounding Sterile Preparations and Guidelines on Handling Hazardous Drugs, 89
ASTM Standard D6978, the *Standard Practice for Assessment of Resistance of Medical Gloves to Permeation by Chemotherapy Drugs*, 25–26
ASTM Standard F739-99a *(Standard Test Method for Resistance of Protective Clothing Materials to Permeation by Liquids or Gases under Conditions of Continuous Contact)*, 26
autoclaves, 37
automated compounding device (ACD), 82
    cleaning of, 119
availability of USP <797>, 1–2

B

Banana Bag, 35
Basics of Aseptic Compounding Technique Videos and Training, 39
beyond-use dates (BUDs), 3, 6, 22, 89
    4-hour, 35
    active pharmaceutical ingredients and other components, 106–107
    biologics, 91
    of chemos, 100
    compounded stock bags, 109–110
    by CSP categories, 102–104
    general information, 99–106
    vial/bag systems, 107
    vials and other dosage forms, 107–109
biological safety cabinet (BSC), 21, 29, 58, 68
biologics, working with, 91
biomechanical engineering, 74
bleach, 117–118
blood components, 91
Board of Pharmacy Specialties (BPS), 14
    Certified Sterile Compounding Pharmacist (BCSCP) certification, 39
bubble point test, 91
buffer rooms. *see* positive pressure buffer rooms
bulk list, 88

C

calculations, 37
calibration, equipment, 75, 79
cameras, 61
cardboard, 59
cefazolin syringes, 91

cellphones, 87
Centers for Disease Control and Prevention (CDC)
    Biosafety in Microbiological and Biomedical Laboratories (BMBL) document, 91
    hand hygiene, 24
    Safe Injection Practices, 33
Certificate of Analysis (CoA), 52, 88, 90
certification and recertification, 5, 80, 83–86, 123–124
Certified Compounded Sterile Preparation Technician™ (CSPT™), 14, 40
Chapter <800> Answer Book, The, 4, 20, 23, 39, 55, 57, 60, 69, 121
chemo
    gloves, 25–26
    gowns, 26–27
chemo rooms, 63, 65, 68–69, 70
    certification of, 85
classified devices, 56
cleaning and disinfecting, 6, 22
    compounding areas, 120–121
    core competencies in, 37
    general information, 113–117
    PECs and other compounding equipment, 118–120
    respiratory protection for, 29
    supplies needed for compounding, 121–122
    types of solutions for, 117–118
cleanroom suites, 61–64, 67–69, 70
    beyond-use dates and, 100
    pass-through chambers to, 71–73
clean side of anteroom, 64, 66
clerkship students, 40
closed system drug-transfer devices, 37
Code of Federal Regulations (CFR), 88
colony-forming units (CFUs), 43, 124, 126, 131
commissioning, 124
community pharmacies, 10
Competence Assessment Tools for Health-System Pharmacies, 15
competence documentation, 15–16, 117
competencies
    core, 37
    hiring personnel with prior, 37
compliance with USP <797>, 9, 11
components
    blood, 91
    conventionally manufactured products as, 6, 51
    core competencies in moving, 37
    nonsterile starting, 51–53, 100
    in nonsterile-to-sterile compounding, 90–92

    policies and procedures for, 21
    receiving and unpacking, 21
    use of conventionally manufactured products as, 6
    use of nonsterile starting, 51–53
Compounded Drug Products That Are Essentially Copies of Commercially Available Drug Products under Section 503A of the Federal Food, Drug, and Cosmetic Act, 11
compounded sterile preparations (CSPs)
    antibiotic, 92, 105
    as components, 6
    elimination of risk levels of, 3
    final checks of, 6
    handling, storage, packaging, shipping, and transport of, 7
    immediate-use (*see* immediate-use CSPs)
    initial training, 37
    intrathecal or epidural, 88, 106
    labeling of, 111–112
    for long-term care (LTC) facilities, 10
    minimum facility requirements for, 55
    presterilization areas for weighing powders, 67
    segregated compounding areas for nonhazardous, 69–70
    time limit for administration of, 11
Compounded Sterile Preparations Pharmacist (BCSCP), 14
compounded stock bags, beyond-use dates (BUDs) of, 109–110
compounding
    activities not considered, 10
    administration distinguished from, 11
    algorithm for determining appropriateness of, 89–90
    allergenic extracts, 7, 36, 76–77, 95
    cleaning supplies needed for, 121–122
    compounding records (CRs), 6, 21, 92–95, 97
    general information, 87–90
    master formulation records (MFRs), 6, 21, 92–93, 96
    nonsterile-to-sterile, 90–92
    policies and procedures for, 21–22
    radiopharmaceuticals, 1, 4, 45, 48, 77–78, 92, 95
    training required for, 15
compounding areas
    allergenic extracts, 76–77
    cellphones in, 87
    cleaning, disinfecting, and applying sporicidal agents in, 6

cleaning of, 120–121
designation of, 21
facilities design for, 55–59
maximum number of personnel in, 87
monitoring of, 20
order of donning garb for, 30
other equipment in, 74–75
policies and procedures for, 20–21
segregated radiopharmaceutical processing areas, 77–78
temperature and humidity requirements for, 57–58
compounding aseptic containment isolators (CACIs), 25, 29, 58, 61, 68
compounding aseptic isolators (CAIs), 25, 47, 58, 61, 66, 68
compounding personnel
initial training for, 37–41
responsibilities of, 15, 21
training of, 15–16, 20
compounding records (CRs), 6, 21, 92–95, 97
Compounding Sterile Preparations, 39
Compounding Sterile Preparations: ASHP's Video Guide to Chapter <797>, 39
computer equipment
cleaning of, 120
tablets, 74
contact lenses, 28
contact plates, 130
containers, sterile, 91
containment segregated compounding areas (C-SCAs), 56, 70–71
surface sampling, 129
containment ventilated enclosure (CVE), 67
contents of sections of USP <797>, 5–8
Controlled Environment Testing Association (CETA), 21, 83
Certification Application Guides (CAGs), 59, 83
conventionally manufactured products, 6, 51
CriticalPoint, LLC, 14, 38

D

daily nonviable monitoring, 79–82
deactivating, 113
decontaminating, 113
dehumidifiers, 81
depyrogenation. *see* sterilization and depyrogenation
designated person, 13–14, 20
dirty side of anteroom, 64, 66

disinfecting. *see* cleaning and disinfecting
dispensing, 10, 111–112
disposable garb, 24
DNV-GL Healthcare, 1
documentation, 7
certification reports, 59
competence, 15–16, 37, 117
training, 38, 40–41
doffing of PPE, 24
donning of PPE, 24, 30
doors, 62
dropper bottles, 91
dry anterooms, 66
dwell time, 114
dynamic conditions, 84

E

earrings, 27
electrolyte bags, 109–110
environmental monitoring
active air sampling, 123, 126–128
general information, 123–126
reacting to out-of-specification results, 131–132
surface sampling, 3, 128–130
Environmental Protection Agency (EPA), 113, 114
epidural CSPs, 88, 106
equipment and supplies, 6
calibration of, 75, 79
cleaning of, 118–120
computer, 74, 120
core competencies in use of, 37
incubators, 47–48, 75, 125–126, 127, 129
other compounding area, 74–75
printers, 64, 74
records of, 21
refrigerator and freezer, 64, 73, 79, 101–102, 105
storage of, 59–60
warming, 74, 105, 125
expiration date, 52–53, 99
Extended Stability for Parenteral Drugs, 39, 106
eyeglasses, 28
eye protection, 28, 113
eyewash stations, 21, 62

F

face shields, 28
facilities and engineering controls, 5. *see also*

primary engineering controls (PEC); secondary engineering controls (SEC)
facility design, 55–59
filtration, 91, 101
Food and Drug Administration (FDA), 1
    503A and 503B lists, 88, 89
    Compounded Drug Products That Are Essentially Copies of Commercially Available Drug Products, 11
    Insanitary Conditions at Compounding Facilities, 134
    List of Drug Products That Have Been Withdrawn or Removed from the Market for Reasons of Safety or Effectiveness, 88
    on what can and cannot be compounded, 88
four hour beyond-use date, 35
freezers, 73, 79, 101–102
fungus, 125

G

garbing, 5, 20, 23–31
    for cleaning, 113
    core competencies in, 37
    eye protection, 28
    general information on, 23–24
    gloves, 20, 25–26
    gowns, 20, 26–27
    hair covers, 20, 27, 30
    masks, 20, 27–28
    procedures for, 29–31
    shoe covers, 20, 28
    sleeve covers, 28
    storage, 57
    training in, 42
general principles of USP <797>, 3–4
Getting Started in Aseptic Compounding, 39
Glossary, USP <797>, 7
gloved fingertip and thumb test, 36, 42–45
gloves, 20, 25–26
goggle, 28, 113
gowns, 20, 26–27
Guide to Parenteral Admixtures, 106

H

hair/head covers, 20, 27, 30
Handbook of Injectable Drugs, 106
hand hygiene, 5, 20, 24–25, 37, 41
hazard communication plans, 16–17

hazardous CSPs, containment segregated compounding areas for, 70–71
hazardous drugs (HDs), 4, 10, 16
    chemo gloves for handling, 25–26
    cleaning supplies for, 121
    containment segregated compounding areas for, 70–71
    decontamination for, 113
    garb for, 23
    minimum facility requirements for, 55
    segregated compounding areas (SEC) for, 58
Hazardous Drugs—Handling in Healthcare Settings: ASHP's Guide to USP Chapter <800>, 39
high efficiency particulate air (HEPA) filters, 58, 62, 68, 69, 83
    in pass-through chambers, 72
    surface sampling, 129
highly pathogenic organisms, 124
high-touch areas, 120
hoods, 55, 56, 60–61, 70, 132
    certifications of, 84–86
    cleaning of, 119
hospital pharmacies, 10
human resources, 13–17
    designated person, 13–14
    documenting competence, 15–16
    hazard communication plan, 16–17
    responsibilities of compounding personnel, 15
humidifiers, 58, 81
humidity requirements and monitoring, 57–58, 59, 62, 64, 79, 80–81

I

immediate use CSPs
    compounded in ambient air, 75–76
    considered compounding, 87
    preparation for administration, 33–36
incubators, 47–48, 75, 125–126, 127, 129
Infection Control Committees, 133–134
infusion time, 99, 102
initial training, 37–41
Institute for Safe Medication Practices' (ISMP)
    Guidelines for Safe Preparation of Compounded Sterile Preparations, 61
International Journal of Pharmaceutical Compounding, 92
International Organization for Standardization (ISO) standards, 56, 68, 70, 72, 77, 78
intrathecal CSPs, 88, 106

intravenous immunoglobulin (IVIG), 91
in-use time, 99
investigational agents, 10
irrigation bottles, 108
IV bags
    beyond-use dates (BUDs) of, 108
    cleaning of, 121–122
IV hoods, 35
IV rooms, 56, 72
    certification of, 84
    cleaning and disinfecting of, 115, 116
    temperature of storage areas outside, 80
IV software systems, 85
IV solutions, 34–36

J

The Joint Commission, 1

L

labeling, 6, 22, 111–112
Lactated Ringers, 36
laminar airflow workbenches (LAFWs), 58, 68
lidocaine preparations, 36
line of demarcation in anterooms, 66
long-term care (LTC) facilities, 10
lot numbers, 94
low-linting disposable towels/wipers, 25

M

mail-order pharmacies, 10
malt extract agar (MEA), 127
mannitol warmers, 48, 125
masks, 20, 27–28, 29
master formulation records (MFRs), 6, 21, 92–93, 96
material safety data sheets (MSDSs), 16
measuring and mixing, 37
media fill test, 36, 46–48
microbiological air and surface monitoring, 5
microbiology departments, 125–126
MINI-BAG Plus, 89, 107
mold, 131–132
monitoring, daily nonviable, 79–82
monthly cleaning, 116, 119
mops, reusable, 114
music, 87

N

N95 respirators, 29
National Formulary (NF) marking, 52
National Institute for Occupational Safety and Health (NIOSH), 16, 26, 29, 57, 60, 63, 70, 121–122
needles, cleaning of, 121–122
negative pressure rooms, 37, 60, 62, 63, 65, 79, 81
    powder hoods in, 85
neonatal total parenteral nutrition (TPN), 109–110
nonhazardous CSPs
    cleaning supplies for, 122
    segregated compounding areas for, 69–70
nonsterile preparations, 1, 10
nonsterile starting components, 51–53, 100
nonsterile-to-sterile compounding, 90–92
nonviable monitoring, 79–82
nuclear medicine departments, 77–78
nuclear medicine technologists, 43, 48
Nuclear Regulatory Commission (NRC), 95
nursing homes, 10

O

Occupational Safety and Health Administration (OSHA), 16, 17
one off compounding, 94
operating room (OR)
    beyond-use dates (BUDs) and prepping for, 108
    OR greens for, 24
out-of-specification results, 131–132
outsourcing facilities, 88
    premixed solutions from, 89
    stock bags from, 110

P

packaging, 22, 111–112
paddles for surface sampling, 129
paper towels, 25
pass-through chambers, 71–73
    air sampling in, 127
    cleaning of, 121
personal hygiene, 5, 20, 24–25, 37
personal protective equipment (PPE), 23
personnel training. *see* training
pharmaceutical manufacturers, 10
    expiration dates, 52–53
    lot numbers, 94

premixed solutions from, 89
vial tops from, 88
pharmacy bulk package (PBP), 109
Pharmacy Competency Assessment Center, 15
Pharmacy Compounding Accreditation Boards, 1
Pharmacy Technician Certification Board (PTCB), 14, 39–40
physician offices, 10
plastic curtains/drapes, 56
policies and procedures, 6, 19–22
positive pressure buffer rooms, 61–64, 65, 68, 79, 81
pass-through chambers to, 72
powder hoods, 85
powders
garb for compounding, 23, 31
presterilization areas for weighing, 67
powered air purifying respirators (PAPRs), 29
power loss, 120
premixed solutions, 89
prepackaging, 11, 89
preparation for administration, 33–34
pressure requirements and monitoring, 59, 62, 64, 79, 81
presterilization areas, 67
primary engineering controls (PEC), 6, 21, 37, 43, 55, 58, 60–61, 67, 80, 83, 85
certification, 123
cleaning and disinfecting of, 115, 118–120
surface sampling, 128–129
printers, 64, 74
probability of a nonsterile unit (PNSU), 91

Q

quality assurance and quality control, 6–7, 22, 133–134

R

radiopharmaceuticals, 1, 4, 45, 48, 92, 95
segregated processing area for, 77–78
reconstitution, 34, 105
refrigerators, 64, 73, 79, 101–102, 105
cleaning of, 121
release inspections and testing, 6, 21
religious head coverings, 27
repackaging, 3, 11
repeater pumps, 82, 84
cleaning of, 119

requalification, 49
respirators, 27, 29
restricted access barrier system (RABS), 68
reusable garb, 24
reusable mops, 114
robots, 60

S

Sabouraud dextrose agar (SDA), 127
safety data sheets (SDSs), 16–17
sampling plan, 124
sanitizing. *see* cleaning and disinfecting
scales, 61
scope of USP <797>, 9–11
secondary engineering controls (SEC), 6, 37, 55, 61–64, 80, 83
certification, 123
segregated compounding areas (SCA), 24, 26, 27, 56, 58, 61–64
allergen extracts preparation in, 76
anterooms for, 66
beyond-use dates and, 100
cleaning and disinfecting of, 114–115
for nonhazardous CSPs, 69–70
order of donning garb for, 30
surface sampling, 129
segregated radiopharmaceutical processing area (SRPA), 77–78
settling plates, 127
shelving, 62, 63, 66
shipping boxes, 59
shoe covers, 20, 28
single-dose ampules, 107
single-dose vials, 107
sinks, 21, 57, 62, 66, 68, 70
sleeve covers, 28
Small Entity Compliance Guide for Employers That Use Hazardous Chemicals, 17
sodium bicarbonate IV, 35
soybean-casein digest media, 47
spills, cleanup of, 29
sporicidal agents, 6, 113, 117
sprinkler heads, 62
stability, drug, 101
standard operating procedures (SOPs), 6, 19–22
sterile containers, 34–35
sterile products and preparations, 1, 3
compounded by students, 87

examples of, 9
general information, 51
initial training for compounding, 37
mixed by nurses for immediate use, 34
nonsterile-to-sterile compounding of, 90–92
receiving areas for, 57
use of nonsterile starting components and, 51–53
see also compounded sterile preparations (CSPs)
Sterile Products Preparation Certificate Program, ASHP, 14
sterilization and depyrogenation, 6
storage areas, 21, 59–60
    in anterooms, 65
    garb, 57
    segregated compounding areas (SEC) used as, 63
    temperature in, 79
supplies. *see* equipment and supplies
surface sampling, 3, 128–130
surfaces and finishes, 59, 62, 63, 67
syringe containers, prepackaging of medications into, 89
syringes, 36, 91
    cleaning of, 121–122
    reconstituted and frozen, 105

T

tape, 67
technician certification, 39–40
temperature requirements and monitoring, 57–58, 59, 62, 64, 79, 80, 101–102, 129
    for shipped products, 112
terminal cleaning, 119
terminal sterilization, 91
TNTC (too numerous to count), 126
total parenteral nutrition (TPN), 109–110
touchscreen monitors, 61
training
    aseptic technique, 45–46
    compounding personnel, 15–16, 20
    designated person, 14
    documentation of, 38
    evaluation and, 5
    garbing, 42
    gloved fingertip and thumb test, 42–45
    hand hygiene, 41
    initial, 37–41

media fill test, 46–48
requalification, 49
trypticase soy agar (TSA), 42, 127

U

UltraTag™, 92
United States Pharmacopeia (USP) marking, 52
United States Pharmacopeia–National Formulary (USP–NF), 101
USP <71> *Sterility Tests*, 47
USP <659> *Packaging and Storage Requirements*, 80
USP <795> *Pharmaceutical Compounding—Nonsterile Preparations*, 1, 3, 10, 95
USP <797> *Pharmaceutical Compounding—Sterile Preparations*, 1
    allergens, 4
    application to animals, 9
    availability of, 1–2
    beyond-use dates (BUDs), 3, 6, 22, 35, 89, 91, 99–110
    certification of engineering controls, 83–86
    cleaning and disinfecting, 6, 22, 29, 37, 113–122
    compliance with USP <797>, 9, 11
    compounding, 87–97
    contents of sections of, 5–8
    daily nonviable monitoring, 79–82
    dispensing and packaging, 10, 22, 111–112
    enforcement of, 11
    environmental monitoring, 123–132
    facility design, engineering controls, and equipment, 55–78
    garb and hand hygiene, 5, 23–31
    general principles of, 3–4
    hazardous drugs, 4
    human resources, 13–17
    immediate use and preparation for administration, 33–36
    list of boxes, 8
    list of tables, 7
    as official standard, 1–2, 9
    personnel training and competence documentation, 37–49
    policies and procedures, 19–22
    quality assurance and quality control, 6–7, 22, 133–134
    scope of, 9–11
    sterile products and supplies, 51–53

where to start with information from, 135–136
USP <800> *Course,* 39
USP <800> *Hazardous Drugs—Handling in Healthcare Settings,* 1, 4, 10, 23, 56, 57, 113
USP <825> *Radiopharmaceutical—Preparation, Compounding, Dispensing, and Repackaging,* 1, 4, 45, 48, 77–78, 92, 95
USP <1113> *Microbial Characterization, Identification, and Strain Typing,* 126
USP <1163> *Quality Assurance in Pharmaceutical Compounding,* 133
USP <1168> *Compounding for Phase 1 Investigational Studies,* 10
USP <1178> *Good Repackaging Practices,* 89
USP *Compounding Compendium,* 92, 101
USP monograph, 96, 99, 101, 105

V

viable monitoring, 79, 123
vial/bag systems, 89
beyond-use dates (BUDs) of, 107
VIAL-MATE, 89, 107
vials
  beyond-use dates (BUDs) of, 107–109
  cleaning of, 121–122
  tops of, 88, 109

W

warmers, 74, 105, 125
washable gowns, 26
waste segregation and disposal, 22
water as component, 52
weekly cleaning, 115
weighing rooms, 67
wet anterooms, 66
windows in pass-through chambers, 72